ENTERIC PARASITES ASSOCIATED WITH HIV/AIDS PATIENTS IN MANIPUR

THE AUTHORS

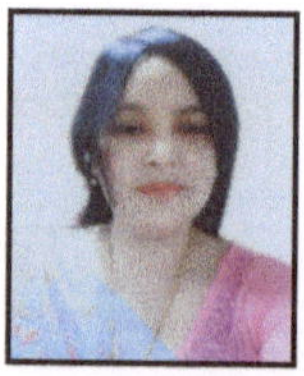

Dr. H. Ranjana Devi, presently working as Post Doctoral Researcher received MSc (Life Sciences, Parasitology) and PhD (Life Sciences, Human Parasitology) from Manipur University. She has worked extensively on the GI parasites associated with PLHA in Manipur and has 08 publications to her credit in journals of national and international repute.

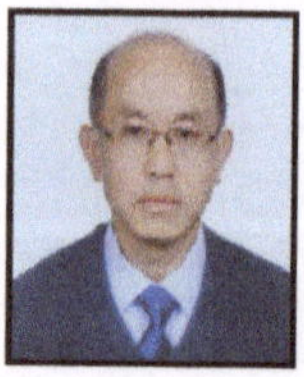

Dr. L. Anand Singh, presently working as Scientist 'C' at Viral Research & Diagnostic Laboratory (VRDL), Department of Microbiology, Regional Institute of Medical Sciences (RIMS), Imphal is an ICMR-NIV (RCVRDL), Pune trained Life Scientist. He was a Fellow of the prestigious Indian Institute of Advanced Study, Shimla (H.P) (2006-2009). He had worked as Research Officer at Molecular Diagnostic Laboratory, Department of Microbiology, RIMS (Imphal) (2010 - 2018). Dr Singh, having a working experience at Defence Research Laboratory (DRDO) Tezpur, Assam (2002-2005), has published 25 original research papers, 01 book and 05 monographs.

ENTERIC PARASITES ASSOCIATED WITH HIV/AIDS PATIENTS IN MANIPUR

H. Ranjana Devi

L. Anand Singh

2025

Scholars World

A Division of

Astral International Pvt. Ltd.

New Delhi – 110 002

ISBN: 9789359195018 (HB)

Published by : **Scholars World**

A Division of

Astral International Pvt. Ltd.

– ISO 9001:2015 Certified Company –

4736/23, Ansari Road, Darya Ganj
New Delhi-110 002
Ph. 011-4354 9197, 2327 8134
E-mail: info@astralint.com
Website: www.astralint.com

In memory of my beloved parents
(Late) H. Devendrajit Singh
and
H. Anandi Devi

ACKNOWLEDGEMENTS

The Almighty God is behind all success, human beings only plan but results are attributed to *Him*; hence my most Pranam to his *Holy Feet* for this humble work.

I express my deep sense of gratitude and indebtedness to my beloved mentor(s) - Dr R. K. Gambhir Singh, Professor, Parasitology Section, Department of Life Sciences, Manipur University; Dr Ng. Brajachand Singh, Professor & former Head, Department of Microbiology, Regional Institute of Medical Sciences and Ex-Dean, School of Medical Sciences, Manipur University and Dr R. Varatharajan, Professor, Entomology Section, Department of Life Sciences, Manipur University for their valuable help, support and encouragement while working as a PhD student and also for critically going through the manuscript.

Acknowledgements are also due to Manipur University and University Grants Commission (UGC) for awarding University Fellowship for pursuing doctoral study.

I also want to keep on record the valuable helps, suggestions, co-operations and unfailing guidance and support from the respected teachers of the Department of Life Sciences, Manipur University in general and Parasitology Section in particular.

I also express my deep and sincere gratitude to the people of the state living with HIV/AIDS and staff of the National Reference Laboratory (NRL) & Molecular Diagnostic Laboratory, Department of Microbiology, RIMS hospital and staff & counsellors working in different drug de-addiction centres located in different parts of the state without whose support, help and co-operation, it would have been not possible to accomplish such a study.

I am also grateful to my husband Dr L. Anand Singh for sharing his creative, scientific, innovative and thought-provoking ideas besides giving physical and moral support and to my loving sons - Laitonjam Dhruv and Laitonjam Dushyant for their understanding and also for making everything worthwhile.

Last but not the least, I express my gratefulness to Astral Publications Pvt Ltd, New Delhi for publishing this piece of research work in the form of a book within a short period of time.

Haodijam Ranjana Devi

Dr Ksh. Birendra Singh, MD
Professor of Medicine
Physician, Anti Retroviral Treatment (ART) Centre (CoE, RIMS)
Member, State AIDS Clinical Expert Panel (SACEP), Manipur
& National Trainer (NACO, GoI)
Department of Medicine
Regional Institute of Medical Sciences,
Imphal – 795 004 (Manipur)

FOREWORD

A number of intestinal parasites thrive in the gastrointestinal tract of HIV/AIDS patient. Infections by enteric parasitic agents constitute a major secondary aggravating factor for these patients, often responsible for worsening the general health condition(s) through the manifestations of gastrointestinal related health problems including diarrhoea, which are sometimes difficult to manage. Moreover, progression and outcome of HIV/AIDS is influenced by various factors such as baseline health, nutritional status, endemic diseases (caused by helminth and protozoan parasites and other microorganisms endemic/ prevalent in that region or area) and access to the therapy. Therefore, it is high time to understand the presentation of HIV disease in the local context by studying the various parasitic diseases prevalent in the region/area and also their association with these patients, if any, because based on these findings, it can be ascertained which parasites are more likely to be frequently acquired by these HIV/AIDS patients as well as which ones are more likely to behave as opportunist parasites.

Identification of parasites associated with HIV/AIDS patients plays a very crucial role in tackling the AIDS epidemic in more effective manner. With better understanding and advanced knowledge on the various aspects of the enteric parasitic infections *vis-a-vis* HIV/AIDS patients, the morbidity and mortality can be reduced/minimized and early diagnosis and prompt treatment will definitely contribute to increased life expectancy among these patients.

I hope this book will help the Life Scientists, Biologists, Zoologists, Physicians and especially the Parasitologists in enlightening and broadening the existing knowledge in this field, especially on GI parasites associated with HIV/AIDS patients of the state.

Prof. Ksh. Birendra Singh

PREFACE

We all are aware that HIV/AIDS patients owing to their immuno-compromised status may harbour a number of pathogenic biological agents/organisms including intestinal parasites. In Manipur, People living with HIV/AIDS (PLHA) are also found to have harboured a number of intestinal parasites. The present book is a humble attempt to bring out a concise, recent and state of the art update on intestinal parasitoses associated with HIV/AIDS community in Manipur - a tiny state situated in the remote northeastern corner of the Indian Subcontinent; a state which is also badly affected by the AIDS pandemic.

We hope, this little piece of work, presented in the form of a book will be useful, informative and help the readers, especially those in the Life Sciences fraternity (Parasitology) in enlightening, enriching and broadening the existing knowledge in this field.

H. Ranjana Devi

L. Anand Singh

CONTENTS

Some Important Technical/Scientific Terms Used in this Book

HIV: Human Immuno-deficiency Virus

AIDS: Acquired Immuno Deficiency Syndrome

HIV positive: An individual who is infected with HIV

HIV negative: An individual who is not infected with HIV

CD_4 count: CD_4 count is the number of CD_4 cells (or helper T cells) present in 1μl of blood.

HIV 1 RNA viral load: It is the quantity of human immuno-deficiency virus (HIV 1 RNA) particles present in an HIV positive individual. It is usually expressed either as number of HIV 1 RNA copies present in 1 ml of blood or as corresponding log_{10} value.

Th 1 cytokine: Small proteinaceous molecules that are released from helper T cell (type 1). It can modulate cell behaviour. e.g. Interleukin – 2

Th 2 cytokine: Small proteinaceous molecules that are released from helper T cell (type 2). It can modulate /activate T - cells, macrophage and dendritic cells.

CV: Calculated value

TV: Table value

df: Degrees of freedom

1

Introduction

Manipur, a small hilly state, is situated in the north eastern border of India. The state covers an area of 22,327sq km, of which the hilly region covers about 91.75%, while the remaining 8.25% of the total geographical area constitutes the central plain/valley region, covering about 1,920 sq.km. The valley is located at an altitude of 790 metres above the mean sea level and the hills at an altitude ranging from 1,500-3,000 metres above the mean sea level. It lies between 23^0 51′ N and 25^0 41′ N latitudes and 93^0 2′ E to 94^0 47′ E longitudes. Generally, two types of climatic conditions are found in this state according to altitude, topography and direction of the prevailing wind system. Tropical monsoon type of climate prevails in the valley area whereas the cool temperate climate prevails in the hilly area. The average maximum temperature of this state is 31^0C while the minimum temperature is 5^0C and the rainfall is about 2,077mm per annum, although rainfall is more in the hills than in the valley or plain region. The type of soil found in the hilly area is red, stony, gravelly or heavy soil with a soil P^H ranging from 5-6 i.e. acidic in nature and in the plain areas, it ranges from sandy loam to clay loam with soil P^H varying from 6.5-8.1. The soil temperature of the state ranges from 18^0C to 32^0C, depending upon topography, soil type and other environmental and geo-climatic factors while the relative humidity of the state varies from 90% to 96% depending upon the seasonal changes, day to day weather condition, geographical variation and type of prevailing vegetation.

According to 2011 census, the total population of the state is 28.56 lakhs, out of which 14.39 lakhs are males and 14.17 lakhs are females. Out of the total population, nearly two third are concentrated in the valley proper and about one third spread over the surrounding hills. 13,31,504 constitute rural population; while 5,05,645 constitute urban population. Scheduled tribes constitute about 6,32,173 of the total population in the state. The valley is inhabited by various ethnic groups, of which, the Meitei constitute the main group in the valley proper while the hills are inhabited by as many as 29 ethnically different tribes, which may be broadly divided into Nagas and Kukis.

Intestinal parasitic infections are common throughout the country with high prevalence rates in many parts of the north eastern states of India. Although the importance of impact of intestinal parasitic infection on the general health of the people has been considerably underestimated, its vital role on the growth and development of people in these regions has been generally accepted. Parasitic diseases affect more than a quarter of the global population and diseases like ascariasis, amoebiasis, trichuriasis and hookworm infection are among the ten most common infections in the world (WHO, 1987).

Parasitic diseases are the cause of more human deaths than anything else apart from HIV/AIDS and TB (WHO, 1999). It has been estimated that about 9 billion people are infected with ascariasis, 5 billion with trichuriasis, 8 billion with hookworm, about 4 billion with amoebiasis, 2 billion with giardiasis (WHO, 1985) and 50-100 million people with strongyloidiasis (Carvalho and DA Fonseca Porto, 2004). As per WHO, at least 2 billion people in the world suffer from helminthiasis and of these approximately 300 million suffer from associated severe morbidity (Savioli *et al.*, 2002). All the more, intestinal worm diseases killed at least 1,35,000 people in 1995 (WHO, 1996). *Ascaris lumbricoides* infection is thought to have caused an estimated 60,000 deaths annually (Montresor *et al.*, 1998).

Malabsorption, diarrhoea, blood loss, retarded growth and impaired working capacity are some of the important health and social problems that result from the infection (WHO, 1981). Apart from morbidity, associated with acute infections, the burden of chronic parasitic infections may affect physical fitness (Stephenson *et al.*, 1990), cognitive performance and educational achievements (Connolly and Kvalsvig, 1992), nutritional status, growth and development (Stephenson, 1994) and school attendance (Nokes and Bundy, 1993). Although children with light infections were thought to suffer no ill effects, there are reports that even low or moderate intensity infection significantly retards childhood growth and development (Stephenson, 1994). As far as the relationship between parasitic infection and their impact on HIV/AIDS patients are concerned, a number of new findings have been published. For instance, helminthic infection influences the HIV disease progression by regulating the host immune response both at cellular and humoral level, as the result of a strong T-helper cell type 2 cytokine (Th 2 cytokine) profile (Bentwich *et al.*, 1996; Kalinkovich *et al.*, 1998; Bentwiz, 1999; Bundy *et al.*, 2000; Borkow *et al.*, 2001; Baum *et al.*, 2003). Parasites like *Strongyloides stercoralis, Ascaris lumbricoides, Trichuris trichiura* and hookworm which are known to be strongly associated with a Th 2 cytokine shift accompanied by eosinophilia could represent a condition associated with rapid immuno-competence deterioration. Parasitization with intestinal worms increases the risk of getting the enteric diseases caused by various microorganisms including *Vibrio cholerae, Salmonella typhimurium* and *Entamoeba histolytica.* Worm infestation can render vaccines useless because the human immune system reacts to worms in a way that is opposite to the response needed to resist diseases caused by viruses like HIV and intracellular bacteria like *Mycobacterium tuberculosis,* the causative agent of tuberculosis (Anon, 2001a). Moreover, inoculation does not protect people against cholera when most of them are infected by worms (Fincham, 2001). Infection with schistosomiasis renders patients more susceptible to infection with HIV-1 (Mwinzi, 2001). HIV can infect cells from people with schistosomiasis more easily and that during co-infection, liver damage (granulomas) due to schistosomiasis is more severe (Mwinzi, 2001).

The presence of *Cryptosporidium parvum* and *Isospora belli* in an otherwise HIV seropositive individual is considered as marker of an immunocompromised status (Bu *et al.,* 1992). The presence of eosinophilia in an individual is generally considered as a marker for worm or parasitic infection and the percent of eosinophilia is considered as a marker of a Th 2 response. Infection with intestinal helminth results in immune responses involving cytokines produced by T-helper cell type 2, with IgE production, eosinophilia and mastocystosis (Bentwich *et al.,* 1996; Kalinkovich *et al.,* 1998; Bundy *et al.,* 2000; Baum *et al.,* 2003). In situations of chronic helminthic infections, the Th 2 subset dominates and is thought to depress T – helper cell type 1 (Th 1) functions, facilitating HIV disease progression (Actor *et al.,* 1993; Bentwich *et al.,* 1996; Borkow *et al.,* 2001; Baum *et al.,* 2003). Th 2 response has been associated with wasting and more rapid HIV disease progression.

Eosinophil percentages are directly and significantly correlated with viral load and inversely correlated with CD_4 (Cluster of Differentiation) cell counts (Actor *et al.,* 1993; Bentwich *et al.,* 1996; Kalinkovich *et al.,* 1999; Borkow *et al.,* 2001). HIV infection is characterized by a Th 1 type immune response and it may result in the decreased interleukin - 5 and IgE responses in patients with strongyloidiasis. Strongyloidiasis usually produces asymptomatic or mild infections but develops into severe disseminated strongyloidiasis in patients with AIDS. The emergence of HIV/AIDS has heightened the spectrum of opportunistic parasites by enabling more aggressive and disseminated parasitic infections in humans, such as cryptosporidiosis, isosporiasis, toxoplasmosis and strongyloidiasis. Individuals with HIV/AIDS infection experience specific immunologic alterations with newly acquired infections or reactivation of latent ones that can occur despite high titres of circulating antibodies. Concurrent infections with ascariasis suppressed immune responses to the oral cholera vaccine. Part of this suppressive effect can be reversed when the patient is dewormed with anthelmintic (Cooper, 2001). Ascariasis in adults affects the immune system in a way that is likely to increase the risk of infection by HIV and tuberculosis. According to Gray (2001), deworming did not influence the HIV viral load of patients. The patients' viral load was as bad before TB medication and deworming as thereafter.

However, Gray (2001) and other workers reported that in patients co-infected by HIV and TB, the infection by any gut parasite was associated with a higher viral load. People who are infected with *Onchocerca volvulus* and other worms are likely to be more susceptible to infection by HIV and that regular deworming could reverse the situation (Sentongo, 2001). According to Wolday *et al.* (2002), treatment of intestinal worms is associated with decreased HIV plasma viral load, however some workers are of the view that treatment of the same has no influence on the plasma HIV viral load and moreover, it is opined that helminthic infection is not associated with faster progression of the HIV disease (Brown *et al.*, 2004). In spite of these views, in recent years, there are reports of decreased HIV plasma viral load when helminth infected patients are treated with anthelmintics. Mulu *et al.* (2013) reported that deworming of intestinal helminths reduced HIV-1 subtype C viremia in chronically co-infected individuals. In India, Ahmad *et al.* (2013) also reported that treatment of parasitic infection in HIV-1 enteric parasite co-infected patients decreased HIV plasma viral load. Walson *et al.* (2008) reported that eradication of *Ascaris lumbricoides* from asymptomatic HIV-1 infected subjects resulted in a significant elevation in CD_4 T cell counts and a trend towards a decrease in the HIV-1 plasma viral load.

It is considered that the possible reason for the decrease of plasma viral load in helminths – HIV co-infected individuals after the deworming of chronically co-infected patients may be due to the decrease of immune activation induced by suppression of parasitic infection. In fact, infection with helminth parasite modulates the host immune response in a specific pattern. The T-helper cell type 2 (also known as Helper T cell type 2) releases the Th 2 Cytokine. This Th 2 cytokine activates T-cells, macrophage and dendritic cells and these chronically activated cells become a favourable site for infection by HIV and for immunosupression by HIV. Ascariasis also activates the release Th 2 cytokine and suppresses the release of Th 1 cytokine. Thus, infection with ascariasis and other soil transmitted helminthiases activate the release of Th 2 cytokine and suppress the release of Th 1 cytokine, i.e., interleukin - 2 and these Th 2 cytokine activated T-cells, macrophage and dendritic cells act as the best niche or site of HIV multiplication and the rate of HIV multiplication is high in these activated cells, resulting in an enhanced disease progression. The T - helper cell type 1 or Helper T-cell type 1 (Th 1) is responsible for the release of Th 1 Cytokine (one of the important Th 1 cytokines being Interleukin – 2). It (i.e., Interleukin - 2) helps in resisting infection by HIV and for resisting progression to AIDS and for anti-HIV vaccine efficacy, because interleukin – 2 increases the level of CD_4 T cells and also restores the immune system. Interleukin is used for the treatment of HIV/AIDS. Not only helminths, but also protozoan parasites are responsible for causing various health related problems in HIV/AIDS patients. These protozoan parasites generally cause diarrhoea. Strictly speaking, diarrhoeal disease is a common illness that affects million of people worldwide and attack rate ranges from 2 to 12 or more illness per person per year (Guerrant *et al.*, 1990). Diarrhoeal diseases mainly affect young children and are also reported to be associated with long term cognitive deficits (Niehaus *et al.*, 2002). An estimated 12,600 child deaths each day is considered to have occurred in Asia, Africa and Latin America due to diarrhoeal diseases

(Guerrant *et al.*, 1990). Irrespective of HIV status, diarrhoea is a common health problem amongst the population of Manipur. Moreover, diarrhoea, either acute or chronic is of common occurrence in HIV infected persons including children. The diarrhoea causing opportunistic parasitic protozoans like *Cryptosporidium parvum, Isospora belli*, etc. are highly prevalent amongst the HIV/AIDS patients of Manipur, whose population is so high in the state that National AIDS Control Organization (NACO) has ranked Manipur as one of the high HIV prevalent states in India. People living with HIV (PLHIV) owing to compromised immune status render them more susceptible to opportunistic infections such as cryptosporidial diarrhoea. Approximately 75% of those with HIV/AIDS are suffering from the problem of chronic diarrhoea and in India, 47% of AIDS patients experienced chronic diarrhoea in 1997, although the spectrum of pathogens involved were not thoroughly investigated (Misra *et al.*, 1998). Moreover, Misra *et al.* (1998) reported that chronic diarrhoea is a major problem in HIV infected adult persons. Diarrhoea rates are 2-6 times higher in PLHIV than in those who are not infected and the rates of acute and persistent diarrhoea are twice as high in population of PLHIV compared to uninfected population (Lule *et al.*, 2005). Diarrhoea reduces the quality of life of people living with HIV (PLHIV) and can speed the progressionfrom HIV to AIDS (WHO, 2010) and there are reports that chronic diarrhoea is also associated with a 3.3 fold increased risk of disease progression (Hira *et al.*, 2003). Moreover, diarrhoeal diseases also reduce the absorption of antiretroviral medicines and essential nutrients (Bushen *et al.*, 2004). WASH (Water, Sanitation & Hygiene) practices such as hand washing, sanitation, water treatment and safe storage have been reported to reduce diarrhoea rate by 30-40% (Curtis & Cairncross, 2003; Fewtrell *et al.*, 2005; Clasen *et al.*, 2007).

In AIDS patients, opportunistic gut infections as well as helminths may cause intestinal disorders by interfering normal absorptive functions of the small intestine (Castello *et al.*, 1996). However, contrasting reports are there regarding the association and impact of parasitic protozoans on HIV/AIDS.

Brown *et al.* (1991) reported that under laboratory conditions, *Entamoeba histolytica* can took up the highly replicative strain of HIV-1. Moreover immunologically detectable HIV-1 was present in the amoebae upto 48 hours after exposure to infected cells, but this virus could not be transferred to uninfected human cells. Amoebae isolated directly from two HIV infected individuals were also found to be positive for HIV-1. However, Burchard *et al.* (1991) reported that no HIV-1 proviral DNA could be evidenced in the *E. histolytica* strains which had been isolated from HIV patients. A soluble protein derived from an invasive strain of *E. histolytica* (amoebic antigen, AA) is reported to be responsible for inducing the replication of HIV. Croxson *et al.* (1988) observed that of the 15 HIV +ve patients, 5(33%) produced HIV P24 (ranging from 31pg/ml to 151 pg/ml) in response to AA in 30-day cell cultures. HIV P24 was expressed in three of seven patients in response to AA, but not to the T-lymphocyte mitogen phytohaemaglutinin. This means certain *E. histolytica* derived specific antigens are responsible for inducing the replication of HIV. Croxson *et al.* (1988) also noted development of AIDS in HIV infected homosexual men after exposure to intestinal parasites. Helminthic infections as mentioned earlier affect more than a third of the world's population and have a similar geographical distribution to that of HIV and tuberculosis (Borkow & Bentwich, 2000). In developing countries like India and in high HIV prevalent states like Manipur, which is socioeconomically backward and geographically isolated, children born in these regions, where endemicity of geohelminth parasites are high, harbour worm most of their lives. Individuals with helminth infections are chronically immune activated and have a very pronounced Th-2 immune profile. Borkow and Bentwich (2000) hypothesized that chronic immune activation and Th-2 immune profile caused by helminthic infections make the host more susceptible to HIV infection and less able to cope with it once infected. They also opined that intestinal helminth infection may also compromise the generation of protective immunity upon vaccination for both HIV and tuberculosis. Borkow and Bentwich (2000) also hypothesized that eradication of helminthic infections may be essential for successful vaccination against HIV and tuberculosis.

India with 1,029 billion population is having an estimated 21,40,000 people living with HIV (PLHIV), out of which 9,08,600 are women (Anon, 2018). Till March 2018, there are 11,81,129 *on ART* patients in this subcontinent (Anon, 2018). India is the country with second highest number of people living with HIV/AIDS next to South Africa till the end of 2002. As far as HIV prevalence is concerned, Manipur has an infection rate greater than 1% and 1.43% adult (15-49 yrs) HIV prevalence has been reported in Manipur (Anon, 2018). In Northeastern India, Manipur has already been identified as one of the states with high HIV prevalence. Since the first report of HIV seropositive patient in Manipur in February 1990, there are 31,549 people living with HIV (PLHIV) in 2017, out of which 14,187 are women (Anon, 2018). A total of 1,612 new HIV infections have been reported in 2017 and till March 2018, there are 12,483 people on ART (Anon, 2018). A total of 1,621 AIDS related deaths have been reported in 2017(Anon, 2018).

Intestinal parasitic infections are prevalent in both non-HIV and HIV infected patients of Manipur. The gastrointestinal parasites prevalent in the HIV/AIDS patients of Manipur include helminths like *Ascaris lumbricoides, Trichuris trichiura, Strongyloides stercoralis,* hookworm, *Enterobius vermicularis, Taenia* sp. and protozoans like *Entamoeba histolytica/Entamoeba dispar, Giardia lamblia, Cryptosporidium* sp., *Isospora belli, Cyclospora cayetanensis* and *Balantidium coli,* etc. to mention a few. Besides these, a number of commensals like *Entamoeba hartmani, Entamoeba coli, Endolimax nana* and *Iodamoeba butschlii,* etc. are also reported to be associated with these immuno-compromised patients (Singh *et al.*, 2004a; Sherpa *et al.*, 2010; Devi *et al.*, 2010; Sarkar *et al.*, 2012). Bundy *et al.* (2000) reported that many of the population at high risk for HIV also live in highly endemic areas of intestinal parasitic infections, which are mainly acquired in childhood and remain as chronic infections into adulthood. The high prevalence of *Cryptosporidium* in HIV/AIDS patients is a serious health concern for these patients, because so far, there is no specific treatment or specific drugs for treating cryptosporidiosis (Inungu *et al.*, 2000; Hunter and Nichols, 2002; Kadappu *et al.*, 2002) and moreover Xiao *et al.* (1999) suggested that persons with AIDS who are also infected with *Cryptosporidium parvum* have a shorter survival time than those with other opportunistic infections.

The situation is more distressing due to the fact that zoonotic transmission of the disease has also been reported recently, thereby increasing the risk of transmitting the animal pathogenic strains to humans. *Cryptosporidium* causes life threatening watery diarrhoea in HIV/AIDS patients and patients with diarrhoea may produce stool volumes that exceed 6 to 17 litres per day (Kreier, 1993). In one aspect, many workers strongly felt it necessary to assess the parasites that are associated with the general population, because intestinal parasitic infections in HIV/AIDS patients depend largely on the prevalence of intestinal parasitism in the local community (Cotte *et al.*, 1993). Even amongst the HIV positive patients, the occurrence of intestinal parasitism differs in between the non-diarrhoeal(s) and patients who experienced diarrhoea. Moreover, the isolation rate of intestinal parasites also varies from region to region and the parasitic agents also differ markedly from one geographical region to another (Sorvillo *et al.*, 1995). Moreover, in addition to the known classical parasites, now-a-days, a group of less known parasitic protozoans, which are generally referred to as opportunist parasites have recently been reported to be associated with HIV/AIDS patients.

Therefore, the importance of these infections in immuno-compromised patients in general and HIV/AIDS in particular cannot be underestimated as *S. stercoralis* infects hundred million people with thousand deaths per year; *C. parvum* infects 40 million people with hundred thousand deaths per year; *I. belli* infects hundred thousand individuals with thousand deaths per year; *G. lamblia* infects 450 million people with thousand deaths annually and *E. histolytica* infects 500 million people with thousand deaths per year (Anon, 2001b).

Thus, visualizing the importance of the impact of the gastrointestinal parasites, on the health of HIV/AIDS patients and with a view to identify the enteric parasites associated with this group of patients, as well as its vital role on the growth and development of people, by and large for a developing country like India and particularly for an economically backward state like Manipur, the present work has been taken up. Thus, assessing the incidence/prevalence, regional endemicity and seasonal prevalence of enteric parasites associated with the HIV/AIDS patients will be of immense value for suggesting effective interventional, management and prophylactic measures for enhancing the quality of life as well as for the well being of the people living with HIV/AIDS (PLHA).

2

A Brief Note on Intestinal Parasites and HIV/AIDS Patients with Special Reference to Manipur

The association of HIV/AIDS patient with a number of different kinds of biological entities including infectious and parasitic agents was reported at the VIIth International AIDS Conference in 1992 (Anon, 1992). Since then, various workers have reported the occurrence of a number of gut or enteric parasites with this group of patients. Castello-Branco *et al.* (1996) reported that opportunist parasitic gut infections cause severe diarrhoea and absorptive dysfunction of the intestine, thereby causing significant mortality amongst the HIV/AIDS patients. Didier *et al.* (1995) found the association of *Cryptosporidium parvum, Isospora belli, Enterocytozoon bieneusi* and *Encephalitozoon intestinalis* with these immuno-compromised patients. The prevalence of *Cyclospora cayetanensis* in these patients were reported by Soave (1996). A number of new findings on parasitoses associated with HIV/AIDS patient were brought to limelight by the research works of various workers and mention can be made of the following investigators like – Brandonisio *et al.* (1987), Hunter *et al.* (1992), Escobedo & Nunez (1999), Inungu *et al.* (2000), Mitarai *et al.* (2001), Fincham (2001), Hunter and Nichols (2002), Kaminskyl *et al.* (2004), Pozio and Morales (2005), Chhin *et al.* (2006), Hosseinipour *et al.* (2007), Bachur *et al.* (2008), Akinbo *et al.* (2010), Cardoso *et al.* (2011), Ram Mohan *et al.* (2013), Darji *et al.* (2013), Zope *et al.* (2014), Chavan and Chavan (2014), Chandra *et al.* (2015), Tin and Wiwanitkit (2015), Patel *et al.* (2015), Vasundhara *et al.* (2015), Eligio - Garcia *et al.* (2016), Adamu and Petros (2016) and Zida *et al.* (2017).

In India, many workers have reported the association of various intestinal parasites with HIV/AIDS patients. Workers like Ayyagari *et al.* (1999), Prasad *et al.* (2000), Bajaj *et al.* (2003), Aggarwal *et al.* (2005) and Attili *et al.* (2006) are some of the north Indian workers who have done remarkable studies with regard to the intestinal parasites associated with HIV/AIDS patients of north India. Ayyagari *et al.* (1999), Prasad *et al.* (2000), Bajaj *et al.* (2003) and Aggarwal *et al.* (2005) reported that *Isospora belli* is the most frequently encountered parasitic agent responsible for diarrhoea followed by *Cryptosporidium parvum* as far as north Indian HIV/AIDS patients are concerned. They also reported the prevalence of non opportunist parasites like *Entamoeba histolytica, Giardia lamblia, Blastocystis hominis, Cyclospora cayetanensis, Ascaris lumbricoides* and *Ancylostoma duodenale*, etc. besides microsporidium like *Enterocytozoon bieneusi*. Prasad *et al.* (2000) reported the prevalence of *Strongyloides stercoralis* in these north Indian patients. Attili *et al.* (2006) reported protozoan parasites like *E. histolytica, C. parvum* and *Isospora belli* besides helminths to have been associated with HIV patients having low CD_4 counts. West Indian workers like Joshi *et al.* (2002) reported protozoans like *Isospora belli, Entamoeba histolytica, Giardia lamblia, Cyclospora cayetanensis* and nematodes like hookworm, *Strongyloides stercoralis* and cestodes like *Hymenolepis nana* besides microsporidia to be prevalent in HIV/AIDS patients of this region.

South Indian workers - Mukhopadhya *et al.* (1999) and Kumar *et al.* (2002) reported a number of parasites to be associated with the HIV/AIDS community of south Indian state (s). The findings and observations as reported by these workers are more or less in conformity with those of the findings of the other Indian workers, working in the different geographical areas/regions of the country.

The occurrence and distributional pattern of intestinal parasitic infection(s) seem to be more or less the same as far as the studies amongst the HIV/AIDS patients from north, west and south Indian states are concerned, except for some slight variation in the incidence/ prevalence of certain individual parasite(s) or species, the reason for which may be attributed to the regional variation that results due to the topographical, climatic and other socioeconomic factors.

CD_4 Count and Intestinal Parasitic Infection

In recent years, various workers have established the relationship between the CD_4 count and the prevalence of intestinal parasitic infection in these immuno-compromised patients. In this regard, mention may be made of workers like Cimerman *et al.* (1999), Blessman & Tannide (2002), Attili *et al.* (2006), Dalvi *et al.* (2006), Sherpa *et al.* (2010), Eligio-Garcia *et al.* (2016), Patel *et al.* (2017) and Tay *et al.* (2017), etc. In immuno-compromised/immuno-suppressed patients like HIV patient, whose CD_4 count is $\leq$ 200 cells per cu. mm. of blood, whenever, a parasite/pathogen infects and colonizes the gastrointestinal tract, it may act as an opportunist and the patient may experience persistent diarrhoea. It has been reported that amoebiasis was associated with HIV patients having a CD_4 range of 28-186; cryptosporidiosis with a CD_4 range of 32-106; isosporiasis with a CD_4 range of 65-70; helminths with a CD_4 range of 125-155 (Attili *et al.*, 2006). Cimerman *et al.* (1999) also reported that infection with *Isospora belli* usually occurs in patients with CD_4 counts less than 100 cells/cu.mm. and instances of this parasite being associated with CD_4 count as low as 64 cells/cu.mm. have been reported. As far as microsporidiosis is concerned, it has been generally accepted that in HIV positive patients whose CD_4 count is between 50 and 100 cells/cu.mm., the probability of suffering from microsporidiosis is very high (Cimerman *et al.*,1999).

In case of cryptosporidiosis, the intensity and duration of diarrhoea is closely associated with CD_4 count. In HIV infected patients with CD_4 count higher than 180 cells/cu.mm., healing of diarrhoea occurs over a period of four weeks, while in patients presenting with more severe immuno-suppression and with a CD_4 count lower than 140 cells/cu.mm., managing diarrhoea and controlling it is a problem and in these conditions patients suffer from persistent diarrhoea (Cimerman *et al.*, 1999).

In northeast India in general and Manipur in particular, few workers have ventured in this field (Sherpa *et al.*, 2010) and it has been reported that intestinal parasitic infections are generally observed in HIV patients having low CD_4 counts.

HIV 1 RNA Viral load and Intestinal Parasitic Infection

In the last few years, various workers (Bentwitz *et al.*, 1999; Feitosa *et al.*, 2001; Wolday *et al.*, 2002; Endeshaw, 2005; Brown *et al.*, 2006; Kassu *et al.*, 2008; Cardoso *et al.*, 2011; Mulu *et al.*, 2013; Eligio-Garcia *et al.*, 2016) have done extensive investigations for establishing the relationship, if any, between the prevalence of intestinal parasitism and HIV-1 plasma viral load in the HIV/AIDS patients.

Endeshaw (2005) reported that most of the opportunist intestinal parasitic diseases like cryptosporidiosis, isosporiasis and intestinal microsporidiosis were found to be associated with high HIV-1 viral load above 10,000 copies/ml. Kassu *et al.* (2008) reported the observation of a relatively high viral load (VL) in patients infected with *Strongyloides stercoralis* ($\log_{10}$ RNA copies/ml: 5.21±0.90, n = 11) and *Entamoeba histolytica* ($\log_{10}$ RNA copies/ml: 5.29±0.58, n = 4). Moreover, Kassu *et al.* (2008) also reported that individuals infected with multiple intestinal parasite species had higher VL than those infected with single parasite, although the difference was not statistically significant. Bentwich *et al.* (1996) and Wolday *et al.* (2002) suggested chronic immune activation caused by infection with intestinal parasites as the main cause for elevated HIV plasma viral load (VL).

Cardoso *et al.* (2011) reported that *Isospora belli* was detected in HIV patients whose viral load was > 1,00,000 copies/ml and *Entamoeba coli* and *Giardia lamblia* were observed amongst individuals with a viral load of 10,000-1,00,000 copies/ml. Cardoso *et al.* (2011) also reported that *Endolimax nana,* the non pathogenic amoeba was observed to be associated with patients having a higher viral load (> 1, 00,000 copies/ml). Mulu *et al.* (2013) reported that chronically HIV-1 serotype - C infected individuals with helminth co- infection have a significantly higher level of HIV viremia compared to helminth uninfected individuals and deworming significantly reduces the level of plasma HIV RNA.

In India, Ahmad *et al.* (2013) had worked on the relationship between the HIV-1 RNA viral load and intestinal parasitic infections.

As far as northeast India is concerned, literature survey shows very scanty, isolated and fragmentary research works on areas pertaining to the enteric parasites associated with HIV/AIDS patients. This does not necessarily mean that HIV/AIDS patients in the northeastern region/states are not suffering from intestinal parasitic infections and other gastrointestinal disorders like diarrhoea but due to the fact that very few workers have ventured in this field of enteric parasitosis, although a number of HIV/AIDS patients of this region are experiencing gastrointestinal related health problems.

In the entire northeastern region, except one report from Assam (Nath *et al.*, 2006), maximum number of workers are encountered in the state of Manipur and no authentic/published report can be traced in case of the other northeastern states. In case of Assam, Nath *et al.* (2006) reported 18.18% of his study group (HIV positive patients) to have experienced diarrhoeal diseases. A well investigated and researched finding is anticipated in this regard, because there are reports that (in HIV/AIDS patients) whenever pathogens are found in the HIV related diarrhoea, protozoan infection dominates over the bacterial causes (Navin *et al.*, 1998; Waber *et al.*, 1999). In Manipur, works pertaining to intestinal parasitic infection associated with HIV/AIDS patients were studied by a number of workers like, Anand *et al.* (1996), Agarwal *et al.* (1998), Anand *et al.* (1998), Singh (1999), Dhanachand and Anand (2003), Singh *et al.* (2004a, 2004b), Devi *et al.* (2010), Sherpa *et al.* (2010), Sarker *et al.* (2012), Kamki *et al.* (2015), Ranjana and Singh (2015), Ranjana *et al.* (2015) and Ranjana *et al.* (2016). As already mentioned, although certain works onprevalence of intestinal parasitic infections associated with HIV /AIDS patients and relationship between CD_4 counts and enteric parasitoses have been initiated, till date literature review reveals no published work pertaining to the seasonal prevalence of these parasitic infections and the relationship between the HIV-1 plasma viral load and that of the intestinal parasitic infections as far as the HIV patients of this state are concerned.

3

Detection and Identification of Parasites (Including Sampling Design)

All the examinations were made in the laboratory. Stool samples were received/ collected mainly from the OPD patients visiting CD_4 count centre and viral load testing centre of the Department of Microbiology, Regional Institute of Medical Sciences Hospital, Imphal, for the hospital based and seasonal prevalence studies, while personal collection was done for the community survey (by arrangement with the MO-in-Charge/Doctor-in-Charge of the various drug de-addiction and rehabilitation centres located in the different districts of the state). The present study was carried out when the state was having only nine districts, i.e. Imphal east, Imphal west, Thoubal, Churachandpur, Tamenglong, Bishnupur, Ukhrul, Senapati and Chandel district. For convenience during the time of study, Imphal east and Imphal west district were clubbed together and studied under a single unit as Imphal district. All the patients/clients involved with this study, as desired by them, were paid some lump sum amount as monetary assistance towards conveyance for bringing the samples/biological specimens.

In situations, where preservation of the stool sample(s) were felt necessary, either 10% formol saline or 2.5 (preferably 4%) potassium dichromate ($K_2Cr_2O_7$) solution or any other appropriate/suitable preservative was used depending upon the nature/type of parasite(s) to be preserved, particular stage(s) of the parasite that is to be observed and investigated later on. Stool samples collected from both the hospital OPD patients (i.e. CD_4 count centre & Viral load testing centre) and the individual patients (from community survey) were then brought to and examined in the Parasitology Laboratory, Department of Life Sciences, Manipur University.

Collection of Sample(s)

a). For hospital based study, a total of 24 samples (a single stool sample was obtained from an individual patient) consisting of 12 males and 12 females were collected every month from the OPD patients (HIV positive) visiting CD_4

count centre & Viral load testing centre, Department of Microbiology, RIMS hospital, Imphal.

b). For community/field based study, samples were collected from the indoor and outdoor patients admitted in the different drug de-addiction and rehabilitation centres located in the different districts of the state. At the time of conducting this study, no definite sample size could be made but was within the range of 35 – 150 patients (only one stool sample was obtained from an individual patient) per district, depending upon the availability of the patient and their willingness to participate in the present study (i.e. participatory tendency).

In case of Imphal district, 300 patients were enrolled for the present study as a large number of patients were interested in participating this study, as they considered the results of the present study would be of immense importance and would help them in assessing their health status with particular reference to the presence or absence of enteric parasitosis. With a view to facilitate data analysis and statistical calculation, the age group was divided into five categories, viz. (10-20) years, (21-30) years, (31-40) years, (41-50) years and 51 years respectively.

Time of collection

Morning stool samples were collected and then transferred to the laboratory, the same day.

Time of Examination

It is not possible to make a correct guess of the time elapsed between the collection and the examination of the stool; however, a limit of six hours can be taken as the maximum.

Type of Stool

Generally the stool sample(s) received for the examination were solid or semi solid (either formed or non-formed) in case of non-diarrhoeal patients while it was in most cases, watery or semi-liquid in case of diarrhoeal patients. Rarely were they hard; in many cases, stool(s) were mixed with washings and/or urine, particularly in females, in which case another sample was sought. Stool samples collected from the full blown AIDS patients were generally watery as only diarrhoeal patients were included under this category.

Detection and Identification of parasites

For the detection and recovery of enteric parasites, a number of different techniques were employed. The identification of intestinal parasites was done as per the standard guidelines of WHO (2001), Cheesbrough (2002), Smith (2002), WHO (2003a, 2003b) and Chatterjee (2011). The standard operating procedures (SOP) of commonly employed techniques are briefly described below:

a. Normal Saline Method (WHO, 2001; WHO, 2003a & 2003b; Chatterjee, 2011)

One drop of 0.9% normal saline is put over a cleaned frosted glass slide (having a thickness of 0.8 – 1mm). Then, a minute portion of the stool is taken with the help of a copper wire loop that has already been sterilized with a Bunsen flame and is placed over the normal saline present on the slide. Then, with the help of the copper wire loop an emulsion is made by mixing the sample with the saline. Then, a glass cover slip (having a technical specification of either No. 1 or 0) is gently and carefully put over it so as to spread out the emulsion into a thin, fairly uniform and transparent layer. Then it is examined under a binocular compound microscope. This preparation is the unstained direct smear.

b. Iodine Wet Preparation Method (WHO, 2001; WHO, 2003a & 2003b; Chatterjee, 2011)

Here, a preparation is made, in which a drop of Lugol's iodine solution (1%) is first added to the drop of saline emulsion and a cover slip (No.0) is then gently placed over it. This particular method is especially employed for the detection of protozoan cyst. In both the above preparations, they were first examined under the low power objective (i.e. 10X & 15X) of the microscope. Starting from one end of the cover slip, the whole slide is carefully scanned and examined. Any suspicious object (if encountered) is centred and focused under the high power objective (40X) for a detailed diagnosis.

c. Formol Ethyl Acetate Concentration Technique (Ichhpujani & Bhatia, 1999; Smith, 2002; WHO, 2003a & 2003b)

The ethyl acetate concentration technique is a specialized parasitological technique for concentrating the cyst/oocyst/egg(s)/ova and larvae of human pathogenic protozoan and helminth parasite(s) that are present in the faecal/ stool sample because it is rapid and can be used to concentrate a wide range of faecal parasites from fresh or preserved faeces. Eggs that do not concentrate well by this technique are those of *Fasciola* species and *Hymenolepis nana*. Occasionally, this technique is also used for the sedimentation and recovery of rhabditiform larva (L_1) of *Strongyloides stercoralis* (besides using the Modified Baermann Funnel Technique) and filariform larva of hookworm. Although, the primary function of this technique is to concentrate the life cycle stage(s) of the parasite, it also facilitates the removal of faecal debris and artefacts present in the stool, thereby making the gross morphology and internal structures of the cyst/egg/ova/larva to be clearly and distinctly visible without much interference and distraction from the pseudo parasites and artefacts of faecal origin. By employing this technique, the risk of laboratory acquired infection from faecal pathogens is minimized as well as it makes the technique safer because the formol saline/formalin will kill the faecal pathogens. When using this technique, cyst(s), oocyst(s), egg(s)/ova and larvae are fixed and sedimented and faecal debris is separated in a layer between the ether and the formol saline while faecal fat is dissolved in the ether.

In this technique, 2 gm of faeces is first emulsified with 10 ml. of distilled water. Then the emulsion is thoroughly stirred with the help of a stirrer or glass rod. Then it is strained through wire gauze having 40-100 meshes to an inch and the filtrate is taken in a 15ml centrifuge tube and is then centrifuged at an RCF (Relative Centrifugal Force) of 750 - 1000 xg (approx. 3000 rpm) for 3 minutes. The supernatant is then discarded and to the sediment, 7 ml of 10% formol saline solution is added. The mixture is then allowed to stand for 10 minutes. To the mixture, 3 ml of ethyl acetate/diethyl ether is added. Then, it is centrifuged again at an RCF of 750 - 1000xg (approx. 3000 rpm) for another 3 minutes, and is allowed to settle. Centrifuging at a particular rpm/rcf and for a time duration other than the prescribed standard value(s) is not generally preferred because, whenever the sample is centrifuged at a higher rpm/rcf value(s) or whenever it is centrifuged for a longer time duration compared to the standard value(s), the rupturing of the helminth egg(s)/ova occurs and on the other hand, centrifuging at a lower rpm/ rcf value(s) or for a shorter time period, results in the lesser detachment of artefacts and debris which are associated with egg(s)/ova and cyst(s) (Smith, 2002), thereby minimizes the chances of recovery, visibility and detection of the cyst/egg(s)/ova and subsequently interferes in the proper identification of the life cycle stage(s) of the parasite.

When the sample is properly centrifuged, four layers appear in the centrifuge tube. They are - a top layer of ether, a second layer consisting of a plug of debris at the interface, a third formol saline layer and a fourth layer consisting of sediment at the bottom.

The debris is loosened with a stick/glass rod and the upper part of the centrifuge tube is cleaned of the fatty debris and then the supernatant fluid is decanted, leaving 3 or 4 drops. The deposit, after shaking is pipette out with a Pasteur pipette to a cleaned glass slide, then a cover slip (No.1) is placed over it and the specimen is examined under the microscope.

It does not cause any distortion of the protozoan cyst(s) or helminth egg(s) and takes a little time in detecting these life cycle stage(s).Then, to a drop of this sediment, one drop of Lugol's Iodine (1%) is added and is examined under the microscope for the detection of protozoan cyst (if any).

The force and the duration of time of centrifugation are important when sedimenting parasites, when performing the formol ether or ethyl acetate concentration technique to sediment faecal parasites. If incorrectly centrifuged, faecal debris may also be sedimented with the parasites. The greater the outward pull due to rotation, i.e. centrifugal force, the more rapid and effective is the sedimentation. Centrifugal force increases with the speed of rotation, i.e. revolutions of the rotor per minute (rpm) and the radius of rotation. The actual sedimentation achieved at a given speed depends on the radius of the centrifuge.

The RCF value is expressed in gravities (g). An RCF (separating capacity) of 1000xg refers to a force 1000 times the force of gravity.

Detection of *Cryptosporidium* and *Isospora*

For the detection of these opportunistic intestinal parasites, the following techniques are employed:

a. Modified Ziehl Neelsen Staining Technique (Neenis, 1992; Smith, 2002; WHO, 2001; WHO, 2003a)

A little portion of the stool sample (either the sample itself, or an emulsion made with normal saline) is taken by a copper wire loop, already sterilized by heating in a Bunsen flame and is then smeared on a clean glass slide (having a thickness of 0.8 to 1mm) and the faecal smear is heat fixed directly over a spirit lamp. Then, 1 per cent cold carbol fuschin is poured over the smeared surface on the glass slide and is then kept for 3 minutes. The slide is then rinsed with tap water. It is then decolourized with 5% HCl (to be prepared from Conc. HCl) or 95% alcohol (Ethanol). During the time, when the decolourization process is underway, the glass slide is occasionally rocked until the colour stops leaching from the slide. The decolourization process is completed within or in less than 15 seconds.

The slide is then rinsed either with distilled or tap water. It is then counterstained with 1 per cent malachite green for 30 seconds. The slide is finally rinsed with distilled/tap water and is then kept in a dust free area so that it is air dried. All the slides were examined for *Cryptosporidium* sp. by using a high powered binocular compound microscope, first with a 40X objective to locate the oocyst(s) and then with a 100X objective to detect the bright red or orange, round or oval structures with a clear halo measuring 3-5 μm in diameter. These were confirmed as *Cryptosporidium* under oil immersion (100X), when the characteristic clear centre with darker periphery or dark centre with light periphery depending on the arrangement of the sporozoites was identified. *Isospora* appears as a characteristically boat shaped oocyst, having a dimension of 35x13 μm with a distinct wall and is readily seen when observed under the 10X objective.

b) Modified Sheather's Sucrose Flotation Technique (Ichhpujani & Bhatia, 1999; John & Petri Jr., 2009)

This technique is employed when the number of excreted oocyst(s) in the stool (as in case of *Cryptosporidium*) is too low and its presence can't be ascertained. Here, faecal sample (approx. 5 gm) is sieved through a cheesecloth or tea strainer to remove the coarse materials.

The sediment is suspended in about 10 volumes of Sheather's sucrose solution (Sp. gr = 1.180). The solution is then centrifuged at 1000 (RCF 300 – 400 xg) -3000 (RCF 750 – 1000 xg) rpm for 2 minutes. After completion of the centrifuge, oocyst will be at the surface of the solution in the centrifuge tube. With the help of a bacteriological loop, oocyst(s) present at the surface of the solution is transferred to a clean glass slide. The slide is then stained with modified Ziehl Neelsen staining method as described above and the slide is then finally examined under the high magnification (100x). This technique may also be used for the detection of cyst/ova of other parasites. This is because of the fact that the specific gravity of helminth ova & larvae and protozoan cyst are in the range of 1.050 to 1.150 and flotation principle utilizes a liquid medium denser than the parasites so that they rise to the surface and can be skimmed from the surface film (Smith, 2002). A successful flotation fluid must not only be heavier than the parasite, but must not produce damaging shrinkage (Smith, 2002).

c) Modified Formol Ethyl Acetate/ Diethyl Ether Oocyst Concentration Technique (Cheesbrough, 2002)

In this technique, 1-2 gm of faecal sample is first emulsified with 4 ml of 10% formol saline by using a glass rod. Here, the faecal sample for the emulsification should be taken from the surface and several places in the specimen. Then, another 4 ml of 10% formol saline is added and is mixed well by shaking. Then it is strained through wire gauze having 40-100 meshes to an inch and the filtrate is taken in a 15ml centrifuge tube. To this filtrate, 3-4 ml of ethyl acetate/diethyl ether is added. Then, the emulsion is thoroughly mixed using either a vortex mixer (for 15 seconds) or stirred with the help of a stirrer or glass rod for 1 minute. After this, loosen the stopper for few seconds to release the pressure that might have been built up inside the centrifuge tube. It is then immediately centrifuged at an RCF of 300 - 400 xg (approx. 1000 rpm) for 1 minute. Using a Pasteur pipette, carefully remove the entire column of fluid below the faecal debris and ethyl acetate/diethyl ether and transfer this to another centrifuge tube. 10% formol saline is then added to make the volume upto 10ml. Now, centrifuge the tube at an RCF of 750 – 1000 xg (approx. 3000 rpm) for about 5 - 10 minutes. The supernatant is then removed and the bottom of the tube is tapped to resuspend and mix the specimen.

The sediment is then transferred to a glass slide having a thickness of 0.8 - 1mm and is examined for the presence of oocyst(s) using 40x objectives.

The modified ethyl acetate/diethyl ether oocyst concentration technique is preferred to Sheather's sucrose floatation technique for concentrating *Cryptosporidium* oocysts because recovery and subsequent staining of the oocysts are better after adopting this technique (Cheesbrough, 2002).

Detection of *Strongyloides stercoralis*

a) Modified Baermann Funnel Technique for the recovery of *Strongyloides* larvae (Ichhpujani & Bhatia, 1999; John & Petri Jr. 2009)

This technique (also known as baermanization) is a specialized technique for recovering the *Strongyloides* rhabditiform larvae present in the stool. The stool may also contain filariform larvae, because while in the lumen of the bowel, they metamorphose into filariform larvae. This technique exploits the tendency of

Strongyloides larvae to migrate from colder to warmer areas. The apparatus used in this technique consists of a glass funnel measuring about 10 cm or greater in diameter and it is set up on a ring stand. The stem of the funnel has a short rubber tube which is provided with a screw clamp.

A round metal sieve or a wire circle of slightly smaller diameter than the top of the funnel is placed over the funnel. Then, two layers of gauze are placed over the round metal sieve. The funnel is then, filled with lukewarm water (42^{0}C) to a level just covering the gauze and an appropriate amount of fresh faeces or stool is placed on the gauze. The stool sample should be placed in such a way that it is partially in contact with the water. The apparatus is left to stand at room temperature for 8-12 hours. The larvae now migrate to the bottom in the fluid. The fluid is then collected in a centrifuge tube, by opening the clamp and a few drops of the fluid is then put either in a cavity block or watch glass for observing the presence of *Strongyloides* larvae under a dissecting microscope or in a cavity slide or glass disc for observation under low power of magnification using a compound microscope. This technique is one of the most sensitive methods for the recovery of *Strongyloides* larvae from the faecal samples.

Observation using Stereoscopic or Dissecting Microscope and High Resolution Compound Microscope

The contents of the sediment, obtained after adopting the ethyl acetate/diethyl ether concentration technique are then transferred to a glass cavity block and are examined under the stereoscopic dissecting binocular microscope (Olympus) for checking the presence of cyst/egg/ova and larvae (especially rhabditiform larva, L_1). Subsequently, the life cycle stage(s) observed (if any), in the cavity block is then carefully pipette out using a pasteur pipette and is placed on a clean 0.8mm/1mm thick frosted glass slide and is then covered with a cover slip (No.0) and is critically examined for the presence of taxonomically important morphological and anatomical characters (if any) using a compound microscope having a high resolving power (Nikon, Eclipse E-200 and Nikon, SMZ 1270). The photomicrograph(s) of the life cycle stage(s) of the parasite(s) and the anterior end and whole specimen in case of *E. vermicularis* were taken using Nikon Eclipse E-200 and Nikon SMZ 1270 microscope. The glass slide having the life cycle stage(s) of the parasite is then carefully transferred onto the stage of a calibrated compound microscope for measurement.

Ocular Micrometry

The dimension(s) of the cyst/egg/ova/larva (if any) are measured using an ocular micrometer in an already calibrated compound microscope (Olympus – 71692). Identification of the parasite(s) was done based on the measurement(s) of the life cycle stages of the parasite(s) as per the standard guidelines (WHO, 2001; WHO, 2003a & 2003b).

Ascaris lumbricoides

Egg/ova:

- Bile stained
- Mammilary coat/layer is present in fertilized corticated egg but absent in fertilized decorticated egg
- Fertilized Egg, L = 55 - 75μm, B = 35 - 50μm.
- Unfertilized egg - rectangular in shape, L = 85 - 95 μm B = 43 - 47 μm.
- Adult parasite whenever obtained/recovered is identified as per the standard guidelines.

Trichuris trichiura

Egg/ova:

- Bile stained, oval/barrel shaped with bipolar mucoid plug, presence of unsegmented protoplasmic mass, L = 50 - 55μm, B = 22 - 24μm.
- Adult parasites (hardly obtained) whenever recovered from the patients are identified as per the standard guidelines.

Enterobius vermicularis

Egg/ova

- Non-bile stained, Planoconvex, L = 50 - 60 μm, B = 25μm.
- Adult female parasite possesses the following characters –
- Presence of cephalic alae
- Presence of oxyuroid type of oesophagus
- Presence of didelphic amphidelphic type of ovary
- L = 8 – 13mm

Strongyloides stercoralis

Rhabditiform larva, the most commonly observed life cycle stage of *S. stercoralis* in the stool/faeces possesses the under mentioned characters:

- Presence of short buccal cavity (4μm)
- Presence of a large genital primordium (22μm)
- Presence of anal pore at a distance of 50μm from the posterior end
- Presence of attenuated tail
- Exhibits whip like movement
- Length = 200 - 250μm, B = 16μm [These parameters are variable]
- Egg and adult parasite(s) are hardly recovered from the stool

Hookworm

Rhabditiform larvae of hookworm exhibit the following characters:

- Presence of a long buccal cavity (15μm)
- Presence of a small genital primordium (7μm)
- Presence of anal pore at a distance of 80μm from the posterior end
- Exhibits snake like movement (glides like a snake)
- L = 250 - 300μm, B = 17μm [These parameters are variable]

Cyst of *Entamoeba histolytica*

- Presence of 1, 2 or 4 nuclei
- Presence of glycogen mass
- Presence of chromatoid bodies with rounded ends
- Cyst dimension, Range = 10 – 20μm, Usual = 12 - 15μm

Cyst of *Giardia lamblia*

- Shows oval shaped structure
- Presence of thick wall
- Presence of 2 – 4 nuclei at one end
- Presence of median bodies
- Cyst dimension, Range = 8 - 19μm, Usual = 10 - 12μm

Oocyst of *Cryptosporidium*

- Presence of bright red/orange round or oval structures with a clear hallo
- Measures 4 - 5μm in diameter

Besides the above mentioned laboratory techniques, a questionnaire survey was also carried out amongst the HIV/AIDS patients who are co-infected with enteric parasites, so that individual specific data/information can be collected from the studied population with a view to assess their socioeconomic status; signs and symptoms frequently reported by these patients due to parasitic infections as well as to ascertain the probable ways/routes of acquiring these infection(s), by designing a proforma containing a wide variety of questions ranging from individual specific parasite related or induced signs/symptoms to the individual specific behavioural and other socioeconomic aspects including food habit, family income, occupation, level of education, standard of living, knowledge of health and hygienic practices, sources of water for drinking and other household purposes, etc. The information thus compiled are then compared and analysed in relation to the laboratory findings to establish and extrapolate relationship (if any) between the socioeconomic/living condition of the patients to that of the acquisition of parasitic infections as well as to study the symptomatology of some of the commonly reported parasitic diseases.

Besides these, statistical analyses (Goon *et al.*, 1987; Beaglehole *et al.*, 1994; Prasad, 1997) are employed wherever necessary by adopting appropriate statistical tools for authentic interpretation of the observations and findings.

4

Intestinal Parasites in HIV Infected Patients of Imphal District

Introduction

HIV positive patients are generally categorized into two groups, i.e. Antiretroviral treatment naive (*ART naive*) and On antiretroviral treatment (*On ART*) patients. *ART naive* patients are those HIV infected patients who are not yet exposed to the anti HIV drugs or who have not enjoyed the antiretroviral treatment and *On ART* patients are those HIV infected patients who are exposed to the anti HIV drugs or who have enjoyed the antiretroviral treatment. It has been reported that incidence or occurrence of intestinal parasites is higher in HIV positive "*ART naive*" patients compared to the HIV positive "*On ART*" patients (Missaye *et al.*, 2013). Moreover, amongst the *ART naive* patients, detection rate of intestinal parasites is more in *ART naive* diarrhoeal patients compared to the *ART naive* non-diarrhoeal patients (Taklemariam *et al.*, 2013).

With a view to assess the occurrence of intestinal parasites in HIV infected patients of Imphal district, a study was conducted in which a total of 300 HIV positive *ART naive* patients were enrolled. There were 200 diarrhoeal (consisting of 100 males and 100 females) and 100 non-diarrhoeal (consisting of 50 males and 50 females) patients. Single stool specimen was collected from each patient for examining the presence of intestinal parasitic infection, if any.

Findings and Analysis

The findings of the above study can be elaborated as follows:

1.1 Prevalence of intestinal parasites in *ART naive* diarrhoeal patients of Imphal District

Out of the 200 HIV seropositive *ART naive* diarrhoeal patients, 31 (15.5%) individuals were found to be infected with various parasitic infections (Table 1.1). While protozoan parasites like *Entamoeba histolytica, Giardia lamblia* and

Cryptosporidium species were prevalent in these diarrhoeal patients, hookworm was the only nematode observed in these patients. Cryptosporidiosis and amoebiasis were the most frequently detected parasitic infection and were observed in each of the 12 (38.7%) patients followed by giardiasis in 6 (19.4%) and hookworm infection in 1 (3.2%) patient respectively (Fig 1.1).

Of the 31 parasite infected patients, there were 18 (58.1%) males and 13 (41.9%) females, however, the difference in sex was not statistically significant ($|z| = 0.976$, $P < 0.05$).

Maximum number of parasite infected patients was observed in the age group of 21-30 years. On X^2 analysis, it was revealed that the age group 21 - 30 years was found to be independent of both the diseases cryptosporidiosis and amoebiasis (In both cases, CV = 0.116, TV = 3.841, df = 1, CV < TV, $P < 0.05$).

On Karl Pearson's correlation coefficient(r) analysis, it was observed that there existed moderate degree of positive correlation between amoebiasis and cryptosporidiosis ($r = 0.6284$).

1.2 Prevalence of intestinal parasites in *ART naive* non- diarrhoeal patients of Imphal District

Of the 100 patients examined for the presence of parasitic infection, only 14 (14 %) individuals were found positive for enteric parasitosis (Table 1.2). The study revealed that the disease amoebiasis was maximum recorded in 8 (57.14%) patients, followed by hookworm infection in 3 (21.42%), trichuriasis in 2 (14.28%) and ascariasis in only 1 (7.14%) patient respectively (Fig 1.2). The occurrence of enteric parasitosis was highest recorded in the 21-30 years age group. Of the 14 parasite positive patients, there were 9 (64.3%) males and 5 (35.7%) females respectively. The difference in sex was found to be not statistically significant ($|z| = 0.86$, $P < 0.05$).

Table 1.1: Prevalence of intestinal parasites in *ART naive* diarrhoeal patients of Imphal district

Total no. of individuals examined (n): 200 No. of individuals found Positive: 31

Parasite(s) detected	No. of individuals found positive in each age group (age in years)									
	5 (10-20)		12 (21-30)		6 (31-40)		7 (41-50)		1 (≤ 51)	
	M	F	M	F	M	F	M	F	M	F
Entamoeba histolytica	1	2	3	2	1	0	2	1	0	0
Hookworm	0	0	0	0	0	0	0	1	0	0
Cryptosporidium species	2	0	3	2	2	1	1	0	1	0
Giardia lamblia	0	0	1	1	1	1	0	2	0	0

Table 1.2: Prevalence of intestinal parasites in *ART naive* non- diarrhoeal patients of Imphal District

Total no. of individuals examined (n): 100 No. of individuals found Positive: 14

Parasite(s) detected	No. of individuals found positive in each age group (age in years)									
	3 (10-20)		4 (21-30)		3 (31-40)		3 (41-50)		1 (≤ 51)	
	M	F	M	F	M	F	M	F	M	F
Entamoeba histolytica	1	0	2	1	0	1	2	0	1	0
Hookworm	0	1	0	0	1	0	0	1	0	0
Ascaris lumbricoides	1	0	0	0	0	0	0	0	0	0
Trichuris trichiura	0	0	0	1	1	0	0	0	0	0

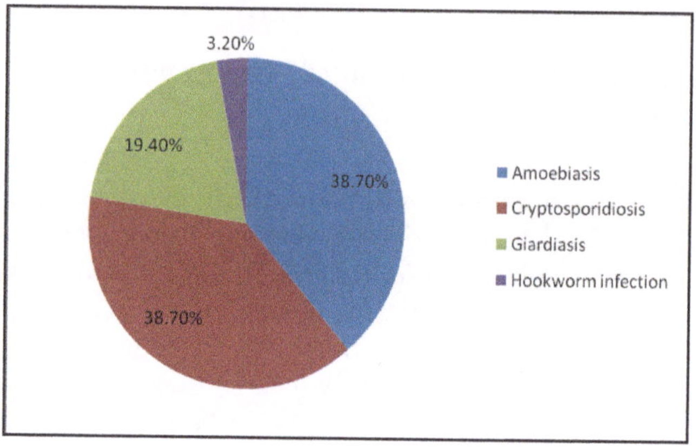

Fig: 1.1: Pie Chart showing distribution of intestinal parasitic infections in *ARTnaive* diarrhoeal patients of Imphal district

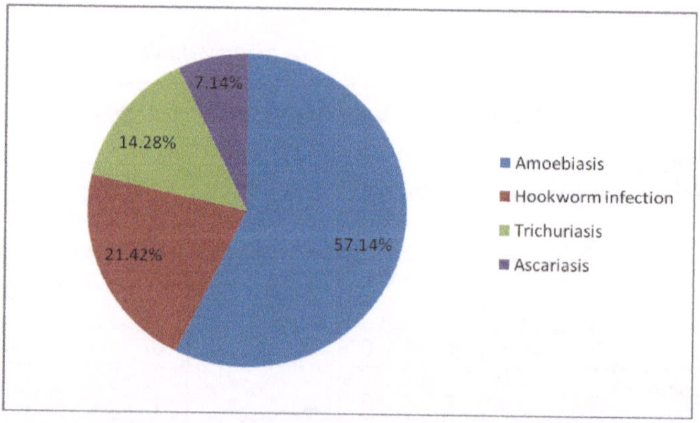

Fig: 1.2: Pie Chart showing distribution of intestinal parasitic infections in *ARTnaive* non- diarrhoeal patients of Imphal district

Discussion

The study revealed that prevalence of enteric parasitic infection was slightly more/higher in the *ART naive* diarrhoeal patients compared to the *ART naive* non-diarrhoeal patients. While the prevalence of enteric parasitosis was 15.5% in the *ART naive* diarrhoeal patients, it was 14.0% in the *ART naive* non-diarrhoeal patients. The present finding of *ART naive* diarrhoeals being more infected with enteric parasites compared to *ART naive* non-diarrhoeals is in agreement with the finding of Taklemariam *et al.* (2013), who also observed higher occurrence of parasitic infections in HIV infected *ART naive* diarrhoeal patients. While three protozoan parasites, namely *E. histolytica, G. lamblia* and *Cryptosporidium* sp. were detected amongst the *ART naive* diarrhoeals; only one protozoan – *E. histolytica* was observed in the *ART naive* non-diarrhoeals. As far as helminth parasites were concerned, while hookworm was the only helminth (nematode) detected amongst the diarrhoeals, three helminths (nematode) namely, hookworm, *T. trichiura* and *A. lumbricoides* were observed amongst the non-diarrhoeals. The study further revealed that while the occurrence of *E. histolytica* was comparatively higher in *ART naive* non-diarrhoeals (n=100), reaching a prevalence rate of 57.14%, a prevalence rate of 38.70% was observed amongst the diarrhoeals (n=200). These non-diarrhoeal patients might have acted as asymptomatic carriers of amoebiasis and most probably it might be one of the reasons for the higher occurrence of this infection amongst them. Similar findings were also reported by earlier workers (Anand *et al.*, 1998). In another finding, while Fontanet *et al.* (2000) reported a higher prevalence of amoebic parasites in HIV patients than in negative patients, Mendez *et al.* (1994) reported a positive association between HIV infection and *E. histolytica*. In case of hookworm infection, it was also observed that its prevalence rate was lowered in the *ART naive* diarrhoeal patients. In both diarrhoeal and non-diarrhoeal patients, the number of infected males exceeds the number of infected females, however, in both the cases, the sex difference was not statistically significant ($P < 0.05$). In both the studies, occurrences of parasitosis were more in the age group 21-30 years. Moreover, none of the patients were recorded to have multiple infections in both the studies.

ART Naive Diarrhoeal Patients

The present finding of cryptosporidiosis being observed in 38.70% of the *ART naive* diarrhoeal patients is more or less within the range as reported by other workers, who based on their studies carried out amongst the HIV positive diarrhoeal patients of Imphal district and other areas in Manipur reported prevalence of this disease within the range of 22.72% to 46.60% of their studied population (Anand *et al.*, 1996; Singh *et al.*, 2004b; Kamki *et al.*, 2015). More precisely, the present finding of 38.70% of the studied population being infected with cryptosporidiosis is in close agreement with the findings of Singh *et al.* (2004b), who reported a prevalence rate of this disease in 36.70% of HIV positive diarrhoeal patients, whose study was carried out at Imphal, Manipur. Moreover, the present finding is consistent with the findings of workers like Lindo *et al.* (1998), Brandonisio *et al.* (1999), Chhin *et al.* (2006), Ajjampur *et al.* (2007) and Kipygen *et al.* (2012), who reported a prevalence rate of this pathogen ranging from 7.7 % to 46 % amongst the diarrhoeal HIV/AIDS patients. The reason for the high occurrence of this disease amongst the studied population might be due to the fact that this pathogen (i.e. *Cryptosporidium* sp.) might have been acquired by these patients through the known transmission routes/mechanisms and the immuno-compromised state of the infected individual boosts up the multiplication and localization of the parasite along its GI tract.

Cardoso *et al.* (2011) and Brandonisio *et al.* (1999) reported giardiasis to be prevalent in 3.50 to 6.10% of their studied population. The present observation of 19.40% of the studied population to be suffering from giardiasis is much higher as compared to the findings of these workers. Moreover, this finding is also much higher compared to the findings of Kamki *et al.* (2015), who reported a prevalence of this disease in 13.63% of his studied group. However, workers like Anand *et al.* (1996, 1998) and Singh *et al.* (2004b) who worked on intestinal parasitosis associated with HIV positive diarrhoeal patients of Imphal district, Manipur, did not report the observation of this parasite in their studied population at the time of their investigation. The occurrence of giardiasis amongst these patients might be due to the acquisition of this parasite by the patients through the consumption and/or drinking of cyst contaminated food or water.

Amoebiasis was also observed in 38.70% of the studied population during the present investigation, however, earlier workers (Singh *et al.*, 2004b; Kamki *et al.*, 2015) did not report the observation of this disease amongst their studied population. The probable reason for the high occurrence of *E. histolytica* might be due to the eating and drinking of quadrinucleated cyst (infective stage) contaminated food and water.

Occurrence of hookworm infection amongst the HIV positive diarrhoeal patients of Imphal district was not reported by earlier workers (Anand *et al.*, 1996; Singh *et al.*, 2004b), however hookworm infection was observed in 3.2% of the studied population during the present study. Although Singh *et al.* (2004b) reported the occurrence of nematodes like *A. lumbricoides, T. trichiura* and *S. stercoralis* amongst the diarrhoeal patients, these parasites were detected in none of the patients during the present study.

ART Naive Non-Diarrhoeal Patients

The present observation of none of the *ART naive* non-diarrhoeal patients to be suffering from cryptosporidiosis is in agreement with the finding of Singh *et al.* (2004b), who based on a study conducted amongst the HIV positive non-diarrhoeal patients of Imphal district reported the non-observance of this disease amongst the studied group. However, the present observation is contradictory to the findings of Anand *et al.* (1998), who reported a 94.4% prevalence of the disease amongst his studied population (asymptomatic patients), which consisted of HIV positive non-diarrhoeal injecting drug users (IDUs). The present observation of 57.14% of the studied population being afflicted with amoebiasis is much higher when compared to the findings of Anand *et al.* (1998), who reported a 5.60% prevalence of this disease amongst the HIV positive non-diarrhoeal patients of Imphal district. However, Singh *et al.* (2004b) reported the non-observance of this disease amongst the non-diarrhoeal HIV seropositive patients of Imphal district.

The present finding of 21.42% of the studied population being infected with hookworm is much higher when compared with the findings of Anand *et al.* (1998) and Singh *et al.* (2004b), who reported a prevalence rate of 1.0% and 6.5% respectively, based on their studies that had been carried out amongst the HIV positive non-diarrhoeal patients of Imphal district.

The present finding of 14.28% of the studied population being infected with trichuriasis corroborates the observations of Singh *et al.* (2004a & 2004b) who reported the prevalence of this disease to be within the range of 9.70% to 21.10%, based on their studies on non-diarrhoeal HIV patients of Imphal district. Previous workers like Anand *et al.* (1998) and Singh *et al.* (2004a & 2004b) based on their studies on HIV positive non-diarrhoeal patients of Imphal district, reported a prevalence of ascariasis ranging from 4.60% to 42.90%. However, in the present investigation, the disease was recorded in only 7.14% of the studied population and this observation corroborates the findings of the earlier workers (Anand *et* al., 1998, Singh *et al.*, 2004a and 2004b) as the presently observed value lies within the range as reported by them. Although Singh *et al.* (2004a & 2004b) reported occurrence of *S. stercoralis* and *E. vermicularis* amongst the non-diarrhoeal patients of Imphal district, none of these parasites were observed among the studied population during the time when this study was carried out.

5

Intestinal Parasites in *ART naive* (diarrhoeal and non-diarrhoeal) Patients of Seven Districts of Manipur

Introduction

Manipur state had only nine (i.e. four valley and five hill) districts when this study was carried out. These districts have varied geo-climatic and environmental conditions due to variation in the topography. In the context of human inhabitation as well as ethnicity, the state has intermingled and multi-ethnicity distribution. The five hill districts are predominantly inhabited by tribal population while the four valley districts are mostly inhabited by Meitei, Tribal and Muslim population. The tradition, custom, standard of living as well as life style of people living in the valley districts have marked difference from that of the ethnic tribal population inhabiting or dwelling the hill regions of the state. Therefore, with the objective of assessing the occurrence of intestinal parasites associated with diarrhoeal and non-diarrhoeal HIV infected *ART naive* patients of the erstwhile seven district (excluding Imphal east and Imphal west district) of Manipur, namely Chandel, Thoubal, Churachandpur, Tamenglong, Ukhrul, Senapati and Bishnupur district, a copro-parasitological study was carried out. For this study, single stool sample(s) from 35 diarrhoeal and 35 non- diarrhoeal HIV infected *ART naive* patients (altogether 70 samples) were collected from each of the seven district of the state. Intestinal parasitic infection associated with diarrhoeal patients of the seven districts of the state are studied and inter-district variation, if any, with regard to the occurrence/distribution of these infections are compared with a view to have a baseline data on the distributional pattern of the gastrointestinal parasites. A similar study was also done in case of non-diarrhoeal patients.

Findings and Analysis

The district wise distribution/occurrence of the intestinal parasitic infection can be summarized as follows:

2.1 Senapati District

Senapati district is situated at the northern side of the state. It is a hilly region and is predominantly inhabited by the Naga tribes.

2.1.1 *ART naive* diarrhoeal patients

Altogether 35 *ART naive* diarrhoeal patients were examined for the presence of intestinal parasitic infections, out of which 14 (40%) patients were found to have been infected with four intestinal parasites (Table 2.1.1). The parasites encountered included two nematodes, i.e. *Ascaris lumbricoides* and hookworm and two protozoans, namely *Cryptosporidium* sp. and *Entamoeba histolytica.* While the parasite *Cryptosporidium* sp. was highest recorded in 7 (50%) patients, parasites like *E. histolytica,* hookworm and *A. lumbricoides* were observed in 4 (28.57%), 2 (14.28%) and 1 (7.14%) patient respectively (Fig 2.1.1). The study revealed that occurrence of parasitic infection was more in 31-40 years age group, and infection rate was higher in males compared to females. Lowest occurrence of parasitic infection was observed in 21-30 years age group. At the time of sample collection, all the parasite positive patients complained of experiencing diarrhoea, on and off, in the preceding two to three months. On X^2 analysis, it was revealed that the disease cryptosporidiosis was independent of the age group 31-40 years (CV=0; TV=3.841; CV < TV, P < 0.05).

2.1.2 *ART naive* non-diarrhoeal patients

In this case also, out of 35 patients examined for the presence of enteric parasitic infections, only 4(11.42%) individuals were found positive for three nematode parasites, i.e. *A. lumbricoides,* hookworm and *E. vermicularis* (Table 2.1.2). While *A. lumbricoides* was observed in 2 (50%) patients, hookworm and *E. vermicularis* were observed in 1 (25%) patient each (Fig 2.1.2).

On X^2 analysis, it was observed that the disease ascariasis was independent of the age group 31-40 years (CV=2.55; TV=3.841; CV < TV, P < 0.05).

2.2 Ukhrul District

Ukhrul district is situated towards the north-eastern side of the state. The region is dominated by the Naga tribe. It is also a hilly region with a low density of population.

2.2.1 *ART naive* diarrhoeal patients

Of the 35 patients examined for the presence of intestinal parasitic infections, 20 (57.14%) individuals were found positive for various parasitic diseases like giardiasis, amoebiasis, strongyloidiasis, ascariasis and hookworm infection (Table 2.2.1). While the protozoan parasites like *G. lamblia* and *E. histolytica* were detected in each of the 5 (25%) patients, nematode parasites like *A. lumbricoides* and *S. stercoralis* were observed in each of the 4 (20%) patients followed by hookworm in 2 (10%) patients (Fig 2.2.1). While the prevalence of parasitic infection was maximum in 31-40 years age group, the age group ≥ 51 years was the least affectedgroup.

2.2.2 *ART naive* non- diarrhoeal patients

Only three nematode parasites were found to be prevalent in the *ART naive* non-diarrhoeal patients of Ukhrul district. These parasites included *A. lumbricoides*, hookworm and *E. vermicularis* respectively (Table 2.2.2).

While 5 (62.5%) individuals were observed to have harboured hookworm, 2 (25%) and 1 (12.5%) patient were found to have been infected by *A. lumbricoides* and *E. vermicularis* respectively (Fig 2.2.2). The age group 31-40 years and 41-50 years were observed to have been more infected.

2.3 Bishnupur District

Bishnupur district is situated towards the south-western side of the state. This district is predominantly inhabited by Meitei although tribal population are there in the interiors of the district.

2.3.1 *ART naive* diarrhoeal patients

During the present study, out of 35 patients examined for the presence of intestinal parasitic infections, 16 (45.71%) individuals were found positive for enteric parasites. The parasite observed included nematodes like hookworm, *Trichuris trichiura* and *A. lumbricoides* and protozoans like *E. histolytica* and *Cryptosporidium* sp. (Table 2.3.1). While amoebiasis and hookworm infection were observed in each of the 5 (31.25%) patients, diseases like ascariasis, trichuriasis and cryptosporidiosis were detected in 1 (6.25%), 2 (12.5%) and 3 (18.75%) patients respectively (Fig 2.3.1). High parasitosis rate was observed in 31-40 years age group. Although maximum number of parasite positive patient belonged to 31-40 years age group, a closer look on the occurrence/incidence of individual parasite species revealed that the age group 41-50 years was maximum parasitized or infected by the sanguinivorous nematode - hookworm. However, on X^2 analysis, hookworm infection was found to be independent of the age group 41-50 years (CV= 2.798; TV= 3.841; CV < TV, P < 0.05).

2.3.2 *ART naive* non diarrhoeal patients

Of the 35 patients, only 5 (14.28%) patients were found to have been positive for parasitic infection. The parasites encountered were hookworm and *E.vermicularis* (Table 2.3.2). While hookworm infection was recorded in 4 (80%) patients, enterobiasis was observed in only 1 (20%) patient (Fig 2.3.2).

2.4 Tamenglong District

Tamenglong district is situated towards the north-western side of the state. It is a hilly region. The district is predominantly inhabited by tribal community, especially Naga. The density of the population is very low and is sparsely distributed.

2.4.1 *ART naive* diarrhoeal patients

Out of 35 patients, 13 (37.14%) patients were found positive for four parasites, namely *S. stercoralis, T. trichiura, G. lamblia* and *Cryptosporidium* sp. respectively (Table 2.4.1). Among the parasite infected patients, there were 8 males and 5 females. Maximum occurrence of the parasitic infection was recorded in 31-40 years age group. In the present study, the disease giardiasis was maximum recorded in 5 (38.5%) patients, followed by cryptosporidiosis in 4 (30.7%), strongyloidiasis in 3 (23.1%) and trichuriasis in 1 (7.7%) patient respectively (Fig 2.4.1). Multiple or mixed infection was observed in none of the patients, as far as the present study is concerned.

2.4.2 *ART naive* non-diarrhoeal patients

Of the 35 patients screened for the presence of enteric parasites, only 4 (11.42%) individuals were found positive for three nematodes, namely *A. lumbricoides, E. vermicularis* and hookworm (Table 2.4.2). While hookworm infection was recorded in 2 (50%) patients, ascariasis and enterobiasis were observed in 1 (25%) patient each (Fig 2.4.2). None of the patients were found to have mixed or multiple infection.

2.5 Chandel District

Chandel district is situated towards the south-eastern side of the state. It is also a hilly region. It is mostly inhabited by the tribal population especially the Naga tribe.

2.5.1 *ART naive* diarrhoeal patients

Of the 35 patients examined for the presence of parasitic infections, 18 (51.42%) individuals were found to have harboured intestinal parasites. These parasites included *S. stercoralis*, hookworm, *G. lamblia* and *E. histolytica* (Table 2.5.1). While the disease amoebiasis was observed in 6 (33.3%) patients; giardiasis, strongyloidiasis and hookworm infection were observed in each of the 4 (22.2%) patients (Fig 2.5.1). Highest occurrence of the parasitic infection was observed in the age group 41-50 years. Amongst the parasite positive patients, none was found to be suffering from mixed or multiple infections.

2.5.2 *ART naive* non-diarrhoeal patients

Of the 35 HIV positive *ART naive* non-diarrhoeal patients examined for the presence of enteric parasitosis, only 6 (17.14%) individuals were found to have been infected with four nematode parasites, viz *E. vermicularis*, hookworm, *A. lumbricoides* and *E. histolytica* respectively (Table 2.5.2).

Occurrence of parasitic infection was more in 31-40 years age group. During the present investigation, the disease amoebiasis and hookworm infection were observed in 2 (33.3%) patients each, while enterobiasis and ascariasis were recorded in 1(16.7%) patient each (Fig 2.5.2).

2.6 Churachandpur District

Churachandpur district is one of the tribal dominated hill districts of Manipur. It is predominantly inhabited by the kukis although there are pockets of Meitei and other tribal communities.

2.6.1 *ART naive* diarrhoeal patients

In the present study, a total of 35 HIV positive antiretroviral (ART) naive diarrhoeal patients were screened for the presence of intestinal parasitic infections. Out of 35 patients, 15(42.85%) patients were found to be positive for parasites like – *Ascaris lumbricoides, Trichuris trichiura, Strongyloides stercoralis, Giardia lamblia* and *Cryptosporidium* sp. (Table 2.6.1). There were 25 male and 10 female patients. Out of 25 males and 10 females enrolled for the present study, 9(36%) males and 6(60%) females were found to be infected with these enteric parasites. None of the patients were found to have mixed infections.

The occurrence of parasitosis was observed to be more in the age group 31-40 years. In the present study, cryptosporidiosis was observed in 5 (33.3%) patients, followed by giardiasis in 4 (26.7%), strongyloidiasis in 3 (20%), ascariasis in 2 (13.3%) and trichuriasis in 1 (6.7%) patient respectively (Fig 2.6.1).

2.6.2 *ART naive* non-diarrhoeal patients

The occurrence of intestinal parasites was less in *ART naive* non diarrhoeal patients compared to the *ART naive* diarrhoeal patient as far as Churachandpur district was concerned. Out of 35 non-diarrhoeal patients examined for the presence of enteric parasites, 11(31.42%) individuals were found to be infected with various parasites like *Ascaris lumbricoides*, Hookworm, *Enterobius vermicularis* and *Trichuris trichiura* respectively (Table 2.6.2). Altogether 23 males and 12 females were examined for intestinal parasitic infection, out of which 8(34.78%) males and 3(25%) females were found positive for the parasitic infections. In the present study, hookworm infection was observed in 5(45.5%) patients, followed by trichuriasis in 3(27.3%), ascariasis in 2(18.2%) and enterobiasis in 1(9%) patient (Fig 2.6.2).

2.7 Thoubal District

Thoubal district is situated towards the southern side of the state. It is a valley region and is inhabited by Meitei, tribal and Muslim communities.

2.7.1 *ART naive* diarrhoeal patients

Of the 35 HIV infected *ART naive* diarrhoeal patients examined for the presence of intestinal parasitic infection, 13(37.14%) individuals were found to have harboured intestinal parasites viz - *Ascaris lumbricoides, Strongyloides stercoralis, Enterobius vermicularis* and *Cryptosporidium* sp. (Table 2.7.1). The disease cryptosporidiosis was maximum observed in 5(38.4%) patients, followed by strongyloidiasis and amoebiasis in each of the 3(23.1%) and ascariasis in 2(15.4%) patients respectively (Fig 2.7.1). None of the patients were observed to have multiple parasitic infections.

2.7.2 *ART naive* non- diarrhoeal patients

A total of 35 non - diarrhoeal individuals were examined and out of which only 9 (25.71%) *ART naive* non - diarrhoeal patients were found positive for three parasites, namely *Ascaris lumbricoides*, hookworm and *Enterobius vermicularis* (Table 2.7.2). While the parasite *A. lumbricoides* was observed in only 1(11.1%) patient, hookworm and *E.vermicularis* were detected in each of the 4 (44.4%) patients (Fig 2.7.2).

Discussion

ART naive diarrhoeal patients

As far as *ART naive* diarrhoeal patients were concerned, highest occurrence of intestinal parasitosis was recorded in Ukhrul district, reaching a prevalence rate of 57.14%, followed by Chandel district (51.42%), Bishnupur district (45.71%), Churachandpur district (42.85%) and Senapati district (40%). The study revealed that the two districts, namely- Tamenglong and Thoubal district recorded the lowest prevalence rate (37.14%) of enteric parasitosis. Literature review reveals publication of one paper (Singh *et al.*, 2004a) that publishes a baseline survey data on the occurrence of intestinal parasitic infections among the HIV patients of three districts of Manipur, i.e. Imphal, Ukhrul and Churachandpur. As far as diarrhoeal HIV patients of Ukhrul district are concerned, although earlier workers (Singh *et al.*, 2004a) reported the occurrence of *A. lumbricoides, T. trichiura* and *Cryptosporidium* in 6.3%, 12.5% and 37.5% of the studied population, the present study reveals the observation of *A. lumbricoides* and hookworm in 20% and 10% of the studied population. Although in the present study, hookworm infection is observed in 10% of the studied population, Singh *et al.* (2004a) did not report the observation of this nematode in their finding. Moreover, while Singh*et al.* (2004a) reported the occurrence of trichuriasis and cryptosporidiosis in his studied population, none of the HIV infected diarrhoeal patients were found tobe suffering from these parasitic diseases as far as the present study is concerned. In case of Churachandpur district, the present finding of ascariasis, trichuriasis and cryptosporidiosis, being prevalent in 13.3% 6.7% and 33.3% of the *ART naive* diarrhoeal patients is comparatively much lower when compared to each of the 23.1% prevalence rates of ascariasis and trichuriasis, 69.2% of cryptosporidiosis as reported earlier by Singh *et al.* (2004a). Although Singh *et al.* (2004a) reported 46.2% of his studied population to be suffering from isosporiasis, none of the patients included in the present study were found to be positive for this opportunistic protozoan parasite.

ART naive non-diarrhoeal patients

Similarly, in case of *ART naive* non-diarrhoeal patients, prevalence of intestinal parasitic infection was maximum in Churachandpur district (31.42%), followed by Thoubal district (25.71%), Ukhrul district (22.85%), Chandel district (17.14%), Bishnupur district (14.28%) and a minimum prevalence of 11.42% was observed in the Senapati and Tamenglong district. In this regard also, earlier workers (Singh *et al.*, 2004a) reported the association of *A. lumbricoides, T. trichiura, E. vermicularis* and hookworm with non-diarrhoeal HIV infected patients of Ukhrul district. However, in the present study, only three nematode parasites namely - *A. lumbricoides, E.vermicularis* and hookworm were found to have been associated with these patients. Both earlier study (Singh *et al.*, 2004a) and the present study revealed a similar observation on the occurrence of *A. lumbricoides, T. trichiura, E. vermicularis* and hookworm among the HIV infected non-diarrhoeal patients of Churachandpur district. However, a low incidence of ascariasis was observed during the present study compared to the earlier finding. In the earlier study, while Singh *et al.* (2004a) reported the prevalence of ascariasis and trichuriasis to the extent of 40% and 10% and enterobiasis and hookworm infection in each of the 5%; a prevalence rate of these parasitic diseases were recorded in 18.2%, 27.3%, 9% and 45.5% of the studied population in the present investigation. In case of ascariasis, the presently observed value is much lower compared to the earlier finding of Singh *et al.* (2004a). On the other hand, for the remaining diseases, i.e. trichuriasis, enterobiasis and hookworm infection, the prevalence rate observed in the present study was higher than those of the earlier reported incidence.

During the study, it has been revealed that occurrence of intestinal parasite appears to be higher in *ART naive* diarrhoeal patients compared to the *ART naive* non- diarrhoeal patients. This observation is in conformity with the findings of Taklemariam *et al.* (2013) who also reported higher occurrence of intestinal parasites in *ART naive* diarrhoeal patients. Sometimes no parasitic agent(s) was detected in HIV infected patients, even though they complained of experiencing diarrhoea. In this regard, it is noteworthy to mention that although parasite(s) can alter intestinal mucosa and cause diarrhoea in patients infected with HIV; there are reports that HIV - the causal organism or aetiologic agent of AIDS, by itself can cause diarrhoea and HIV induced enteropathy (Eligio-Garcia *et al.*, 2016). Moreover, in some cases, ART treatment may cause this symptom (i.e. diarrhoea) as a side effect of ART drugs. Therefore, caution should be taken in establishing the cause of diarrhoea and the relation between enteric parasitic infection and presence of diarrhoea because in HIV infected patients, presence of diarrhoea is not necessarily an indication or marker for the presence of enteric parasitic infection. On the other hand, patients who did not experience diarrhoea were also occasionally found to have harboured intestinal parasites.

Table 2.1.1: Prevalence of intestinal parasites in *ART naive* diarrhoeal patients of Senapati district

Total number of individuals examined = 35 Number of positive individuals = 14

Parasite(s) detected	No. of individuals found positive in each age group (age in years)									
	0 (10-20)		2 (21-30)		6 (31-40)		3 (41-50)		3 (≥ 51)	
	M	F	M	F	M	F	M	F	M	F
Ascaris lumbricoides	0	0	0	0	0	1	0	0	0	0
Hookworm	0	0	0	0	1	0	1	0	0	0
Cryptosporidium sp	0	0	1	0	2	1	0	1	1	1
Entamoeba histolytica	0	0	1	0	1	0	0	1	1	0

Table 2.1.2: Prevalence of intestinal parasites in *ART naive* non-diarrhoeal patients of Senapati district

Total number of individuals examined = 35 Number of positive individuals = 04

Parasite(s) detected	No. of individuals found positive in each age group (age in years)									
	0 (10-20)		1 (21-30)		2 (31-40)		1 (41-50)		0 (≥ 51)	
	M	F	M	F	M	F	M	F	M	F
Ascaris lumbricoides	0	0	1	0	0	0	1	0	0	0
Hookworm	0	0	0	0	1	0	0	0	0	0
Enterobius vermicularis	0	0	0	0	0	1	0	0	0	0

Table 2.2.1: Prevalence of intestinal parasites in *ART naive* diarrhoeal patients of Ukhrul district

Total number of individuals examined =35 Number of positive individuals = 20

Parasite(s) detected	No. of individuals found positive in each age group (age in years)									
	0 (10-20)		5 (21-30)		8 (31-40)		5 (41-50)		2 (≥ 51)	
	M	F	M	F	M	F	M	F	M	F
Ascaris lumbricoides	0	0	1	0	2	1	0	0	0	0
Hookworm	0	0	0	1	0	0	0	1	0	0
Strongyloides stercoralis	0	0	1	0	2	0	0	1	0	0
Giardia lamblia	0	0	0	1	1	1	2	0	0	0
Entamoeba histolytica	0	0	1	0	0	1	1	0	1	1

Table 2.2.2: Prevalence of intestinal parasites in *ARTnaive* non-diarrhoeal patients of Ukhrul district

Total number of patients examined = 35 Number of positive individuals = 08

Parasite(s) detected	No. of individuals found positive in each age group (age in years)									
	0 (10-20)		1 (21-30)		3 (31-40)		3 (41-50)		1 (≥ 51)	
	M	F	M	F	M	F	M	F	M	F
Ascaris lumbricoides	0	0	0	0	0	0	1	1	0	0
Enterobius vermicularis	0	0	0	0	0	1	0	0	0	0
Hookworm	0	0	1	0	1	1	1	0	1	0

Table 2.3.1: Prevalence of intestinal parasites in *ARTnaive* diarrhoeal patients of Bishnupur district

Total number of individuals examined =35 Number of positive individuals = 16

Parasite(s) detected	No. of individuals found positive in each age group (age in years)									
	0 (10-20)		5 (21-30)		6 (31-40)		5 (41-50)		0 (≥ 51)	
	M	F	M	F	M	F	M	F	M	F
Ascaris lumbricoides	0	0	0	0	1	0	0	0	0	0
Trichuris trichiura	0	0	0	0	1	1	0	0	0	0
Entamoeba histolytica	0	0	2	1	0	1	0	1	0	0
Cryptosporidium sp	0	0	1	0	1	0	1	0	0	0
Hookworm	0	0	0	1	1	0	2	1	0	0

Table 2.3.2: Prevalence of intestinal parasites in *ARTnaive* non-diarrhoeal patients of Bishnupur district

Total number of individuals examined = 35 Number of positive patients = 05

Parasite(s) detected	No. of individuals found positive in each age group (age in years)									
	0 (10-20)		1 (21-30)		3 (31-40)		1 (41-50)		0 (≥ 51)	
	M	F	M	F	M	F	M	F	M	F
Hookworm	0	0	1	0	1	1	1	0	0	0
Enterobius vermicularis	0	0	0	0	0	1	0	0	0	0

Table 2.4.1: Prevalence of intestinal parasites in *ART naive* diarrhoeal patients of Tamenglong district

Total number of individuals examined = 35 Number of positive individuals = 13

Parasite(s) detected	No. of individuals found positive in each age group (age in years)									
	0 (10-20)		4 (21-30)		6 (31-40)		2 (41-50)		1 (≥ 51)	
	M	F	M	F	M	F	M	F	M	F
Strongyloides stercoralis	0	0	1	0	1	1	0	0	0	0
Trichuris trichiura	0	0	0	0	0	0	1	0	0	0
Giardia lamblia	0	0	1	1	1	2	0	0	0	0
Cryptosporidium species	0	0	1	0	0	1	1	0	1	0

Table 2.4.2: Prevalence of intestinal parasites in *ART naive* non-diarrhoeal patients of Tamenglong district

Total number of individuals examined = 35 Number of positive individuals = 04

Parasite(s) detected	No. of individuals found positive in each age group (age in years)									
	0 (10-20)		1 (21-30)		2 (31-40)		1 (41-50)		0 (≥ 51)	
	M	F	M	F	M	F	M	F	M	F
Ascaris lumbricoides	0	0	0	0	0	1	0	0	0	0
Enterobius vermicularis	0	0	0	1	0	0	0	0	0	0
Hookworm	0	0	0	0	1	0	0	1	0	0

Table 2.5.1: Prevalence of intestinal parasites in *ART naive* diarrhoeal patients of Chandel district

Total number of patients examined = 35 Number of positive individuals = 18

Parasite(s) detected	No. of individuals found positive in each age group (age in years)									
	0 (10-20)		4 (21-30)		5 (31-40)		6 (41-50)		3 (≥ 51)	
	M	F	M	F	M	F	M	F	M	F
Giardia lamblia	0	0	1	1	0	0	1	1	0	0
Hookworm	0	0	0	1	0	2	1	0	0	0
Entamoeba histolytica	0	0	1	0	2	0	1	1	1	0
Strongyloides stercoralis	0	0	0	0	0	1	1	0	1	1

Table 2.5.2: Prevalence of intestinal parasites in *ART naive* non-diarrhoeal patients of Chandel district

Total number of patients examined = 35 Number of positive individuals = 06

Parasite(s) detected	No. of individuals found positive in each age group (age in years)									
	0 (10-20)		2 (21-30)		3 (31-40)		1 (41-50)		0 (≥ 51)	
	M	F	M	F	M	F	M	F	M	F
Ascaris lumbricoides	0	0	0	0	1	0	0	0	0	0
Hookworm	0	0	0	0	1	0	0	1	0	0
Enterobius vermicularis	0	0	0	1	0	0	0	0	0	0
Entamoeba histolytica	0	0	1	0	0	1	0	0	0	0

Table 2.6.1: Prevalence of intestinal parasites in *ART naive* diarrhoeal patients of Churachandpur district

Total number of patients examined = 35 Number of positive individuals = 15

Parasite(s) detected	No. of individuals found positive in each age group (age in years)									
	1 (10-20)		5 (21-30)		6 (31-40)		1 (41-50)		2 (≥ 51)	
	M	F	M	F	M	F	M	F	M	F
Ascaris lumbricoides	0	0	0	1	0	1	0	0	0	0
Strongyloides stercoralis	0	0	1	0	1	1	0	0	0	0
Cryptosporidium sp.	0	1	1	0	1	1	0	0	1	0
Gardia lamblia	0	0	1	0	1	0	1	0	1	0
Trichuris trichiura	0	0	0	1	0	0	0	0	0	0

Table 2.6.2: Prevalence of intestinal parasites in *ART naive* non- diarrhoeal patients of Churachandpur district

Total number of patients examined = 35 Number of positive individuals = 11

Parasite(s) detected	No. of individuals found positive in each age group (age in years)									
	3 (10-20)		3 (21-30)		3 (31-40)		1 (41-50)		1 (≥ 51)	
	M	F	M	F	M	F	M	F	M	F
Ascaris lumbricoides	0	0	1	0	1	0	0	0	0	0
Hookworm	1	0	1	0	1	0	0	1	0	1
Enterobius vermicularis	1	0	0	0	0	0	0	0	0	0
Trichuris trichiura	1	0	0	1	1	0	0	0	0	0

Table 2.7.1: Prevalence of intestinal parasites in *ART naive* diarrhoeal patients of Thoubal district

Total number of patients examined = 35 Number of positive individuals = 13

Parasite(s) detected	No. of individuals found positive in each age group (age in years)									
	2 (10-20)		4 (21-30)		3 (31-40)		3 (41-50)		1 (≥ 51)	
	M	F	M	F	M	F	M	F	M	F
Ascaris lumbricoides	0	0	0	1	1	0	0	0	0	0
Strongyloides stercoralis	0	0	1	0	1	0	1	0	0	0
Entamoeba histolytica	0	1	0	1	0	0	1	0	0	0
Cryptosporidium sp	1	0	1	0	0	1	0	1	1	0

Table 2.7.2: Prevalence of intestinal parasites in *ART naive* non- diarrhoeal patients of Thoubal district

Total number of patients examined = 35 Number of positive individuals = 09

Parasite(s) detected	No. of individuals found positive in each age group (age in years)									
	0 (10-20)		5 (21-30)		3 (31-40)		1 (41-50)		0 (≥ 51)	
	M	F	M	F	M	F	M	F	M	F
Hookworm	0	0	2	0	1	0	1	0	0	0
Enterobius vermicularis	0	0	1	1	1	1	0	0	0	0
Ascaris lumbricoides	0	0	0	1	0	0	0	0	0	0

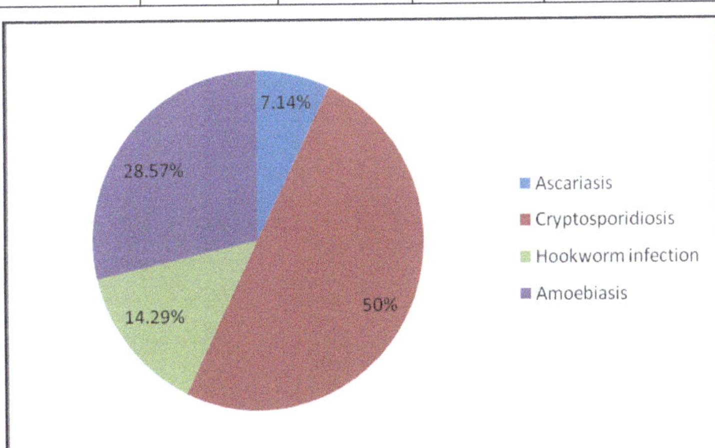

Fig 2.1.1 Pie chart showing the incidence of intestinal parasitic infections among *ART naive* diarrhoeal patients of Senapati district

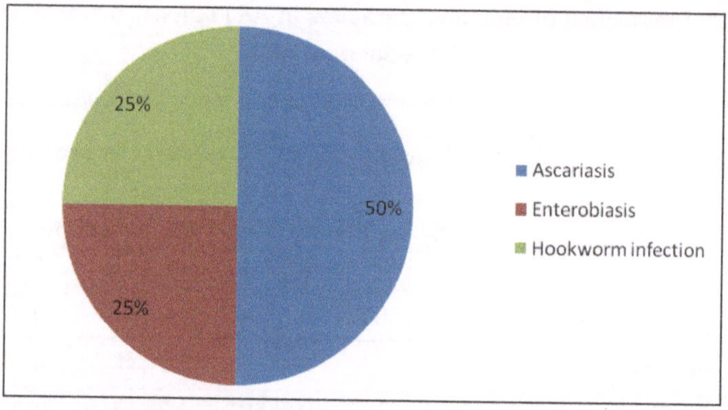

Fig 2.1.2 Pie chart showing the incidence of intestinal parasitic infections among *ART naive* non-diarrhoeal patients of Senapati district

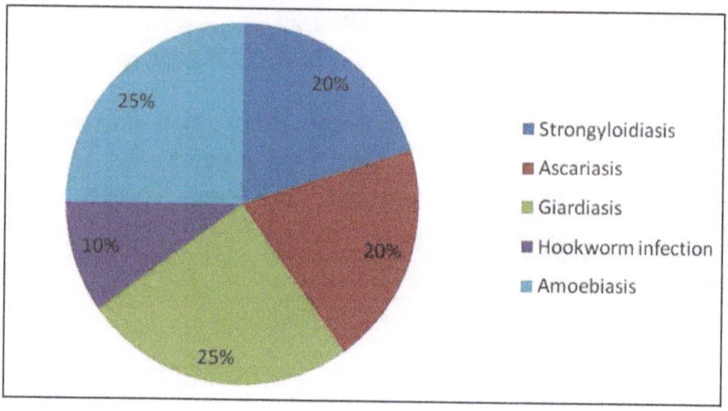

Fig 2.2.1 Pie chart showing the incidence of intestinal parasitic infections among *ART naive* diarrhoeal patients of Ukhrul district

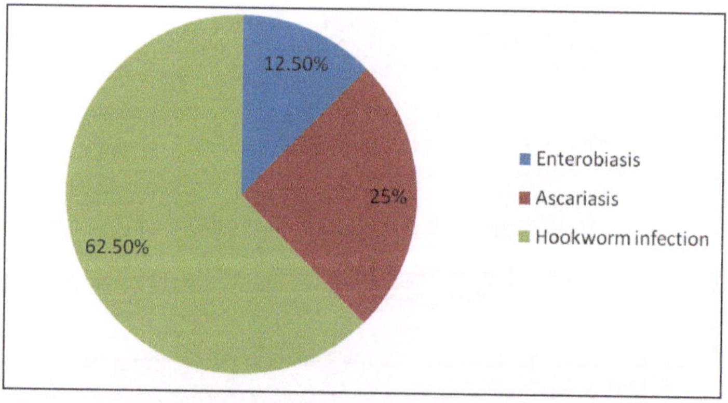

Fig 2.2.2 Pie chart showing the incidence of intestinal parasitic infections among *ART naive* non-diarrhoeal patients of Ukhrul district

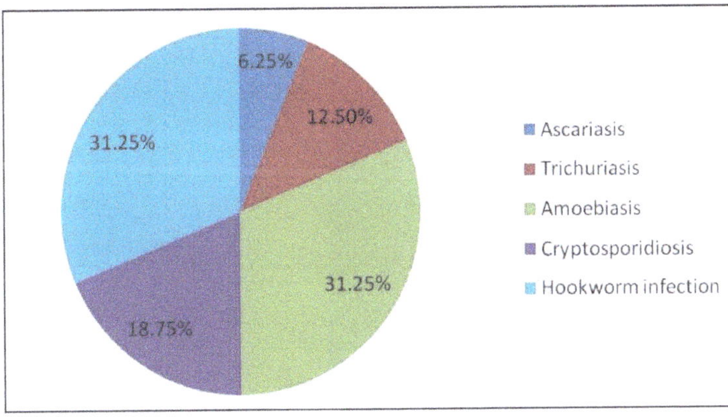

Fig 2.3.1 : Pie chart depicting the incidence of intestinal parasitic infections among *ART naive* diarrhoeal patients of Bishnupur district

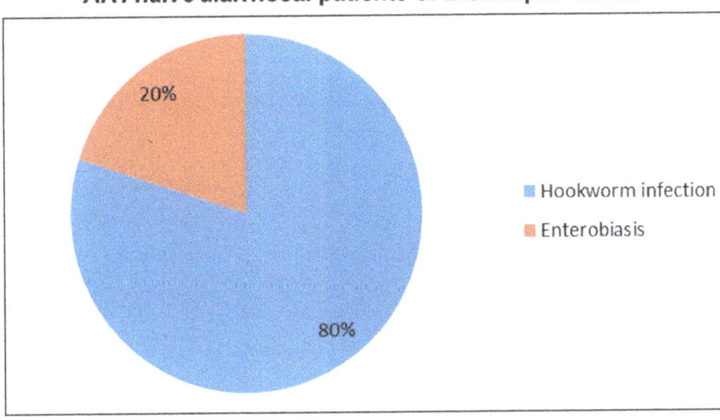

Fig 2.3.2: Pie chart depicting the incidence of intestinal parasitic infections among *ART naive* non-diarrhoeal patients of Bishnupur district

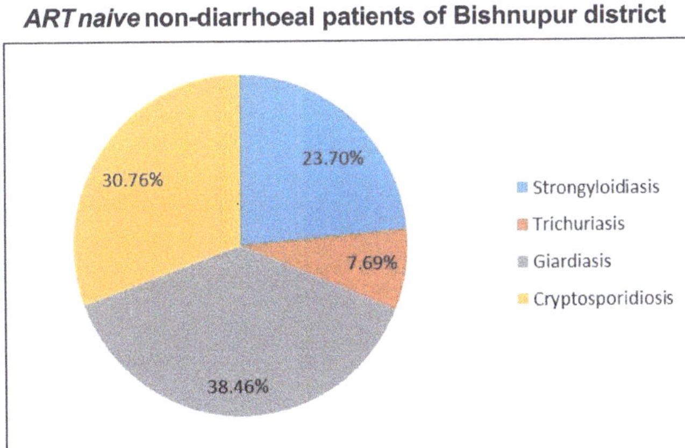

Fig 2.4.1 Pie chart depicting the incidence of intestinal parasitic infections among *ART naive* diarrhoeal patients of Tamenglong district

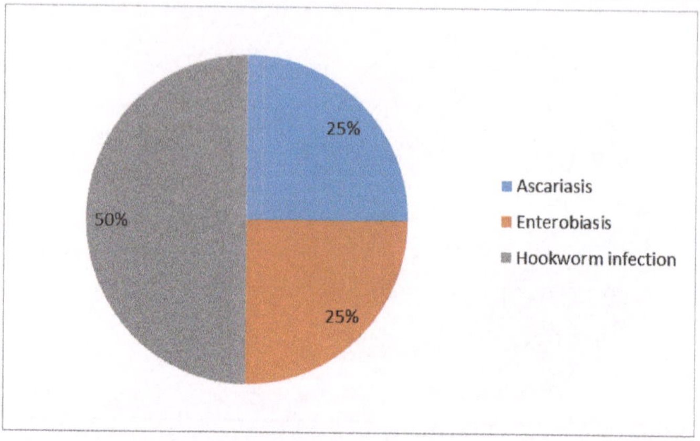

Fig 2.4.2: Pie chart depicting the incidence of intestinal parasitic infections among *ART naive* non-diarrhoeal patients of Tamenglong district

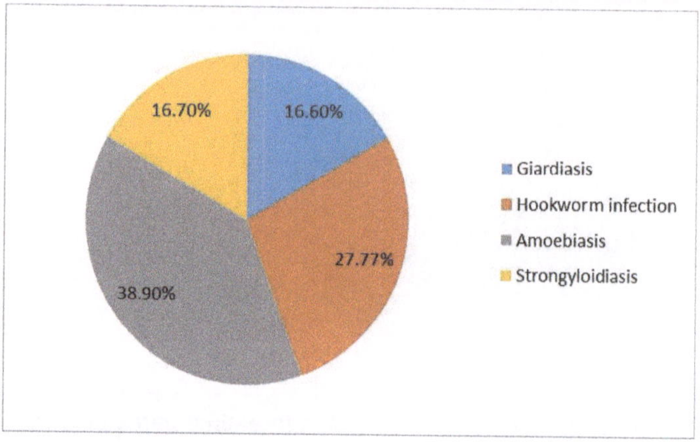

Fig 2.5.1: Pie chart depicting the incidence of intestinal parasitic infections among *ART naive* diarrhoeal patients of Chandel district

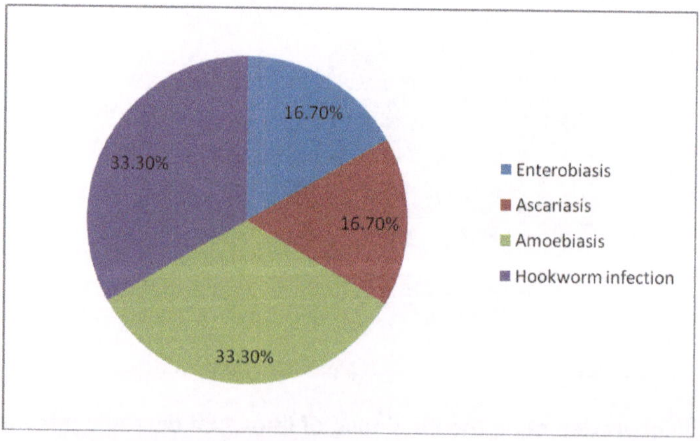

Fig 2.5.2 Pie chart depicting the incidence of intestinal parasitic infections among *ART naive* non-diarrhoeal patients of Chandel district

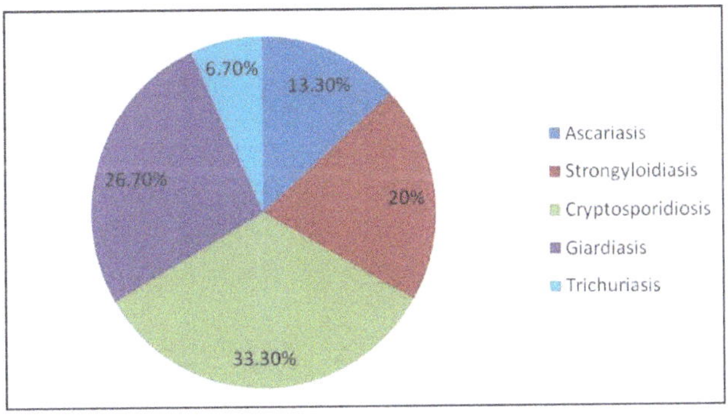

Fig 2.6.1 Pie chart illustrating the incidence of intestinal parasitic infections among *ART naive* diarrhoeal patients of Churachandpur district

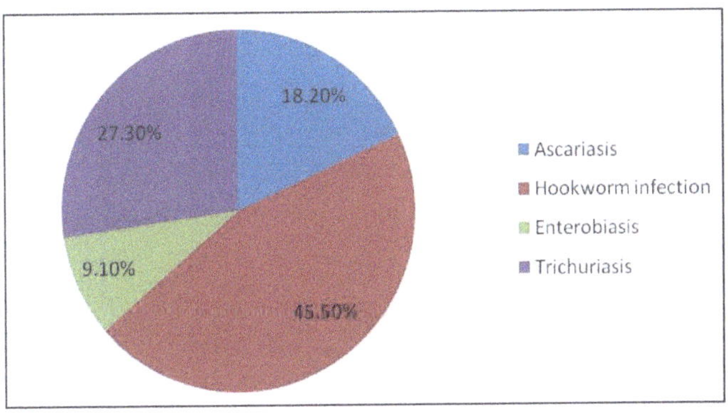

Fig 2.6.2 Pie chart illustrating the incidence of intestinal parasitic infections among *ART naive* non-diarrhoeal patients of Churachandpur district

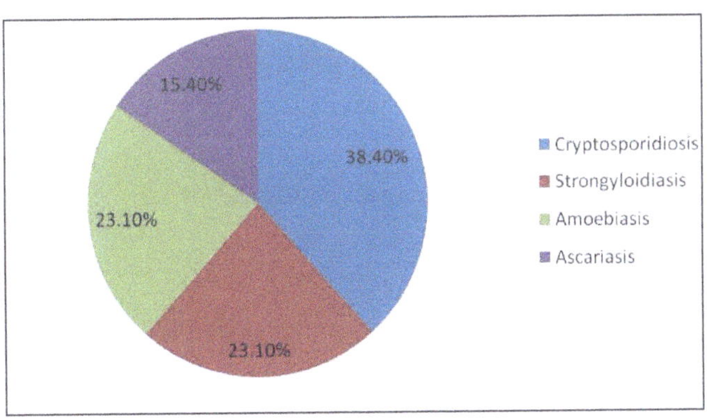

Fig 2.7.1 Pie chart illustrating the incidence of intestinal parasitic infections among *ART naive* diarrhoeal patients of Thoubal district

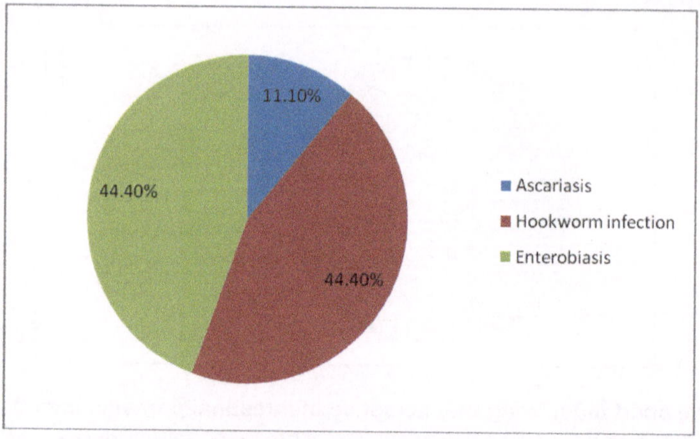

Fig 2.7.2 Pie chart illustrating the incidence of intestinal parasitic infections among *ART naive* non-diarrhoeal patients of Thoubal district

6

Seasonal Prevalence of Intestinal Parasites Associated with HIV/AIDS Patients of Imphal District

Introduction

Occurrence, endemicity and seasonal prevalence of parasitic diseases are influenced by environmental factors. Irrespective of the immunological status of the host or individual, repeated or continuous exposure to the infective stage of the parasite increases the risk of acquiring the infection. In this regard, continuous or persistent occurrence of the infective stage of a parasite or parasite itself, in a particular geographical area or region is more or less influenced by the prevailing geo-climatic condition of that particular area/region, which, in turn, favours the endemicity of the disease. Physical environmental factors like temperature, rainfall, humidity and soil type etc. are known to affect the prevalence of intestinal parasitic infections (May, 1958; Misra, 1970; Howe, 1977). Bhattacharya *et al.*, (1985) also reported that prevalence of intestinal parasitic infection is influenced by both physical environmental factors and the socio cultural factors. Majumder *et al.*, (1984) based on a study in West Bengal, reported differences in the prevalence of intestinal parasitism between and within northern sub Himalayan and southern coastal ecological zones. In north-eastern states of India in general and Manipur in particular, literature review reveals very few published or researched works pertaining to the seasonal prevalence of enteric parasitic infections associated with HIV patients. Previous workers had worked in this regard and reported the prevalence of parasitic diseases like ascariasis, trichuriasis, hookworm infection, amoebiasis, isosporiasis, and cryptosporidiosis amongst the HIV infected patients of Manipur irrespective of their HIV treatment status (whether *ART naive* or *On ART*) (Anand, 1999; Dhanachand & Anand 2003). Moreover, variation in the occurrence and seasonal prevalence of selected intestinal parasitic infections *vis – a – vis* environmental factors like temperature, rainfall and humidity had also been reported (Anand, 1999).

Therefore, with a view to study the seasonal prevalence of intestinal parasitic infections in *ART naive* and *On ART* patients & their co-relationship with certain physical environmental factors, this study was carried out during two years' period.

In the first phase, which was conducted during the period of January to December 2014, occurrence of parasite(s) amongst the HIV infected *ART naive* patients were monitored throughout the year. In the second phase, occurrence of the parasite(s) associated with the HIV infected *On ART* patients were assessed during the period of January to December 2015. During the two years' study period, a total of 576 samples (288 samples from *ART naive* patients during Jan - Dec 2014 & 288 samples from *On ART* patients during Jan - Dec 2015) were collected from the patients visiting CD_4 count (FACS unit) centre and Molecular Diagnostic Lab (HIV-1 viral load testing centre) of the Department of Microbiology, Regional Institute of Medical Sciences (RIMS), Imphal. A total of 24 (consisting of 12 males and 12 females) first morning passaged unpreserved stool samples were collected per month from the patients residing/living in the Imphal district for this study (irrespective of age, ethnicity, religion, marital and health status).

Findings and Analysis

The findings of the above work are described below under different sub-headings:

A. Seasonal prevalence of intestinal parasitic infection associated with *ART naive* patients of Imphal District (January – December 2014)

Nematodes like *Ascaris lumbricoides, Trichuris trichiura,* Hookworm, *Enterobius vermicularis, Strongyloides stercoralis* and protozoans like *Cryptosporidium* sp, and *Entamoeba histolytica* were observed in the HIV infected *ART naive* patients of Imphal district during the period of January – December 2014 (Table 3.1). The disease ascariasis, caused by *Ascaris lumbricoides* was recorded in only five months of the study period (Fig. 3.1.1). Maximum prevalence of the disease was observed in August (16%) followed by April (12.5%) and June (8.3%). The disease was not evident during the remaining months of the study period. In majority of the patients, bile stained fertilized corticated egg/ova was the most frequently observed life cycle stage of the parasite; while fertilized decorticated egg/ova and unfertilized corticated egg/ova were observed in few of the patients. Adult parasite was recovered from two patients during the period of study. The number of egg/ova observed per slide ranged from 11 to 25. The disease trichuriasis, caused by *Trichuris trichiura* was also found to be associated with the *ART naive* HIV infected patients of Imphal district (Fig. 3.1.2). Although a prevalence rate of 8.33% was observed in the month of April, only 4.16% was recorded in January and June. The bile stained barrel shaped egg having two mucoid plugs, was the predominantly and frequently detected life cycle stage of the parasite. Adult parasite was neither detected nor recovered in none of the infected patients. The number of egg/ova observed per slide ranged from 8-12.

The disease hookworm infection was more or less prevalent throughout the year (Fig. 3.1.3). The highest prevalence of the disease was observed in August, reaching a peak value of 16%, followed by 12.5% (April and June) and 8.3% (March) respectively. Infection rate was higher in males (60%) compared to females (40%). Most of the patients were asymptomatic and the vermiform rhabditiform larva (L_1 stage) was the most frequently observed life cycle stage of the parasite as far as the present study was concerned. It was also found to be associated with those samples, the examination of which was deferred or delayed for about 3-5 hours and occasionally in those patients who complained of experiencing chronic watery diarrhoea. The number of egg/ova observed per slide ranged from 8-15, while the number of rhabditiform larvae observed per slide ranged from 15 to 25.

The disease enterobiasis, caused by *Enterobius vermicularis* was also one of the enteric parasitic infections found to be associated with the *ART naive* HIV infected patients of Imphal district (Fig. 3.1.4). During the study period, the disease was maximum observed in the month of July (12.5%) followed by January and August (8.33% in both the months), and subsequently by May and September (4.16% in both the months). Infection rate of the disease was comparatively higher in females (89%) than in males (11%). The partially embryonated egg/ova was the most frequently observed life cycle stage of the parasite when adhesive cellophane tape method (WHO, 2003a) was employed. It was also occasionally observed in the stool samples. Gravid female was recovered from the perianal region of three female patients.

The disease strongyloidiasis, caused by *Strongyloides stercoralis* was also found almost throughout the year (Fig. 3.1.5). The highest prevalence of this disease was observed in July reaching a peak value of 12.5% and the lowest prevalence of the disease was observed in the months of January, March, and November each showing a prevalence rate of 4.16%. Of the 10 patients found positive for the disease, there were 4 males (40%) and 6 females (60%) respectively. The most frequently observed life cycle stage of the parasite was rhabditiform larva (L_1 stage) and the number of rhabditiform larvae observed per slide ranged from 5 to 36 approximately. All the patients complained of loose watery intermittent diarrhoea, at the time of sample collection.

The disease amoebiasis, caused by *Entamoeba histolytica* was more or less uniformly prevalent throughout the year (Fig 3.1.6). High occurrence of the disease was recorded during May, October, and November, with a prevalence rate of 16% in each of these months while lowest prevalence of the disease was observed in the months of March, August and September, with a prevalence rate of 4.16% in each month. The occurrence of the disease was more in males (52%) compared to females (48%). The most frequently observed life cycle stage of the parasite was tetra-nucleated (quadrinucleated) and binucleated cyst. Trophozoite was also observed in very few of the samples collected from the patients. The number of the cysts observed per slide ranged from 6 to 15, depending upon the individual patient.

The protozoan *Cryptosporidium* sp was also observed to have been associated with these patients throughout the year (Fig 3.1.7), although the patients complained of severe diarrhoea or loose motion infrequently. Most of the patients complained of intermittent diarrhoea of low intensity and short duration, which resolves spontaneously or sometimes in certain cases after taking medication. In many of the patients who had experienced watery diarrhoea, due to cryptosporidial infection, the frequency and severity of the diarrhoea varies greatly as the health status of the individual varies. The highest prevalence of the disease was observedin the month of July (33.33%), followed by February and September (12.5% in each),while minimum prevalence rate of 4.16% each was recorded during the period ofMarch, August and October respectively. The disease was more prevalent among the males (62%) compared to females (38%). The number of oocyst(s) observed perslide was ≥10.

B. Seasonal prevalence of intestinal parasitic infection associated with *On ART* patients of Imphal District (January – December 2015)

Parasitic protozoans like *Cryptosporidium* sp., *Entamoeba histolytica, Giardia lamblia* and nematodes like hookworm was found to be prevalent in the HIV infected *On ART* patients of Imphal district during the period from January to December 2015 (Table 3.2).

The disease cryptosporidiosis was observed amongst the studied population during April, July and October only, showing a prevalence of 4.16% in each of these months (Fig. 3.2.1). These patients were observed to have excreted oocysts of the parasite in small numbers ranging from 3 to 6 oocysts/ slide. These patients also complained of chronic intermittent diarrhoea during the period of the study.

The disease amoebiasis was also observed amongst the studied population. The disease was maximum recorded in the month of July, reaching a peak value of 8.33% (Fig. 3.2.2). A prevalence rate of 4.16% were recorded during the remaining months of the year except the five months of January, February, April, October and December during which no positive case was observed. The life cycle stage(s) of the parasite occasionally observed amongst these patients were the tetra nucleated or quadrinucleated cyst and to a lesser extent the trinucleated cyst and precyst. The number of cyst observed per slide ranged from 16 to 20.

The disease giardiasis was detected amongst the patients in the months of April, July and August (Fig. 3.2.3). A prevalence rate of 4.16% each was recorded in the months of April and July, while a highest prevalence of 8.33% was observed in the month of August. The most frequently observed life cycle stage of the parasite was the cyst. The number of cysts observed per slide ranged from 3 to 7. All the parasite positive patients complained of loose motion or watery diarrhoea, at the time of sample collection.

The disease hookworm infection was observed in the HIV/AIDS patients who had complained of abdominal discomfort and mild diarrhoea. The parasite was recorded amongst the HIV patients having a rural setting. The disease was prevalent in June, August, September and December (Fig. 3.2.4), however a higher incidence rate of 8.33% of the disease was observed in the months of September and December respectively. All the patients were found to suffer from mild infection and none of the patients were anaemic rather healthy. Although few egg/ova were detected at the time of coprological examination, rhabditiform larva (L_1 stage) was the predominantly observed life cycle stage of the parasite. The number of larvae observed per slide range from 5 to 12.

Discussion

The prevalence of a particular parasite species varies, as its occurrence/ distribution or endemicity is more or less influenced by the seasonal variations as well as the changes/fluctuations in the geoclimatic/environmental setting of a particular region or area. Altogether there were 89 parasite positive *ART naive* patients, out of which 44 were males and 45 were females. Altogether 30.9% of *ART naive* patients were found to be positive for a number of enteric parasites. In the present study, the number of parasite positive males and females were almost the same and there was no statistically significant sex differences ($|z| = 0.12859$; $P< 0.05$). On Karl Pearson's correlation coefficient (r) analysis, it was observed that possibly no correlation existed between the diseases hookworm infection and amoebiasis ($r = -0.1805$); hookworm infection and cryptosporidiosis ($r = -0.1728$) and also in between the disease amoebiasis and cryptosporidiosis ($r = -0.0467$). Although there was possibility of positive correlation between cryptosporidiosis and that of the temperature ($r = +0.4441$) and humidity ($r = +0.4010$), possibly no correlation existed between the disease and rainfall ($r = +0.1660$). Moreover, possibly no correlation was also evident between amoebiasis and that of the temperature ($r = -0.0163$), rainfall ($r = -0.2787$) and humidity ($r = -0.2066$).

In the present study, a moderate occurrence of the parasites like *Ascaris lumbricoides, Trichuris trichiura,* and *Entamoeba histolytica* were observed amongst the *ART naive* patients who had come from those areas/localities where access to the basic health amenities like availability of safe drinking water supply and other hygienic facilities are either poor or lacking. In fact, the probable reason for the prevalence of parasitic infections amongst the *ART naive* patients residing in these areas might be due to a number of factors. These factors might have included besides unavailability of safe drinking water supply, that of unhygienic and unhealthy practices, low standard of living, lack of knowledge of health education and/or negligence/ ignorance of basic health and sanitation guidelines towards maintaining a neat and clean surrounding or environment in and around the place of living. In the present study, the probable reason for the high occurrence of strongyloidiasis may be due to its opportunistic nature, potentiality to induce auto infective cyclesand immuno-compromised condition of the patient besides the known extrinsic and intrinsic factors that may facilitate the acquisition of the disease. Moreover, the patients who were diagnosed as suffering from strongyloidiasis were mostly farmers (engaged with fishery/ piggery/poultry/ cattle rearing) or vegetable growers, who by virtue of their occupation, were at high risk of acquiring these infections while working in their respective work place (s) including paddy fields and vegetable fields.

The occurrence of the diseases like hookworm infection and cryptosporidiosis may also be due to the known transmission mechanisms as mentioned above. In case of enterobiasis, since the infective stage of the parasite, i.e. the partially embryonated egg/ova is airborne; acquisition of the infective stage might have occurred through inhalation of the airborne egg/ova over and above the known transmission mechanisms.

In the present study, most of the pinworm positive patients were found to have lived in congested houses, which might have facilitated the transmission of the disease. In this study, *G. lamblia* was observed amongst the *on ART* patients only and these patients might have acquired the disease through the known transmission mechanisms.

The prevalence of intestinal parasitic diseases(s) and especially of food- and water- borne infection(s) shows considerable variations in distribution and seasonal occurrence between the different countries as well as within the same country due to the influence of geographical and climatic factors (WHO, 1981). Ascertaining seasonal variation in infection is important as the time frame in which transmission occurs in a specified area can indicate a more appropriate time for the treatment of population by mass chemotherapy and also help to predict outbreaks of infection and plan more effective control measures.

Generally, climatic factors particularly humidity and temperature have always had a relationship to water borne diseases and strictly speaking, several factors may contribute to the high prevalence of soil transmitted helminth (STH) infection viz, soil type, amount of rainfall, temperature, humidity and other sociobehavioural variables (Belding, 1965). In fact advent of rainy season marks the beginning of many infectious, diarrhoeagenic and communicable food- and water- borne diseases including enteric parasitic infections.

Warm and moist environment facilitates the survival of Ascaris eggs with moisture making more eggs viable and infective (WHO, 1964; Crompton & Pawlowski, 1985). Rainfall provides the essential moisture for eggs survival.

An increase in transmission during the rainy months is most probably due to these reasons. The scattering and sorting action of rain (Brown, 1927; Beaver 1975) can effectively disperse and transport eggs/ova over long distances. Ascaris eggs can also percolate to deeper strata of the soil due to the leaching effects of rain (Brown, 1927; Storey & Phillips, 1985), leaving fewer eggs on the soil surface. The lower rates of transmission during the hot drier months is due to the fact that eggs exposed to sunlight during summer became desiccated rapidly and died depending partly upon the type of soil and humidity, moreover, exposure to tropical heat and sunlight may reduce the persistence of these eggs on the soil surface (Wong and Bundy, 1990).

It has been demonstrated that exposure to direct sunlight (28° C to 42° C) for 7 or more hours render the helminth eggs (especially that of *Ascaris*) non-infective. Heavy rainfall is more likely to disperse the eggs horizontally and vertically. A steady rainfall throughout the month would help maintain the required moisture making more eggs viable and infective. Temperature range of 18-28°C is optimal for the maturation of the helminth egg/ova to become infective in soil (Belding, 1965). Moist soil is also favourable for helminth ova development and maturation (Belding, 1965). Although moist soil is favourable for the helminth ova development and maturation, a conducive temperature within the range of 18-28°C and especially of a minimum of 18°C is optimal for the maturation of helminth egg/ova in the soil. This temperature (18-28°C) also favours the development of ascaris and trichuris ova into infective stage in the soil.

In fact, this temperature facilitates the transformation of non-infective egg/ova of *Ascaris lumbricoides* to that of the egg containing second stage juvenile, which is the infective form of the parasite. The fertilized eggs of *A. lumbricoides* become infective or infectious after two weeks in soil and they can persist in soil for 10 years or more. Ascaris eggs are also highly resistant to dryness and temperature fluctuation (Hunter *et al.*, 1976).

Besides the above mentioned factors, it has been generally accepted that in HIV/AIDS patients, the immuno-compromised state of the infected individuals boost up the multiplication and localization of the parasites along its gastrointestinal tract.

As far as *ART naive* patients were concerned, although samples for the study were obtained from them, irrespective of their health status (CD_4 cells count and presence of other opportunistic infections like TB, oral candidiasis, etc.) and particularly of the fact whether they experienced diarrhoea or not, it was revealed that parasite occurrence rate was higher in *ART naive* diarrhoeal patients compared to *ART naive* non diarrhoeal patients. The present finding is more or less in agreement with the findings of Taklemariam *et al.*(2013), who also observed that parasite prevalence was significantly higher in HIV infected *ART naive* diarrhoeal patients.

As far as *On ART* patients were concerned, as they had already been treated with ART drugs which are considered to have lethal or deleterious effect(s) on the viability/survivality of luminal parasites, whether intracellular or extracellular, the occurrence and/or prevalence of intestinal parasitism was much reduced in these patients.

Moreover, there are reports that low prevalence of these endoparasites may be linked to highly active antiretroviral therapy (HAART) since antiretroviral therapy can change the profile of parasite infections, probably because of the reconstitution of cell immunity and action of these drugs on parasites (Bachur *et al.*, 2008), even in those individuals with no specific therapy for enteric parasites (Oldfield, 2002). Altogether, there were only 21(7.29%) parasite positive patients. It consisted of 12 males and 9 females respectively. The parasites encountered in this group of patient included *G. lamblia, Cryptosporidium* sp., *E. histolytica* and hookworm. The present observation of higher occurrence of enteric parasitosis among the *ART naive* patients compared to *On ART* patients is in consistent with the findings of Missaye *et al.* (2013), who based on a study conducted in Northwest Ethiopia, also reported higher prevalence of enteric parasites in patients who do not receive ART treatment. In the present investigation, prevalence of parasitic infection is higher in the *ART naive* patients compared to the *On ART* patients, even though the intensity of infection/parasite burden is light or low in the *ART naive* patients.

However, the occurrence of *Cryptosporidium* is higher in *ART naive* diarrhoeal patients. In fact, the low intensity of the infection may be due to the inter-species competition. Since the causal organism of diarrhoea in HIV infection may include a variety of bacterial, viral and protozoal agents, further studies are needed to know whether organisms other than presently encountered parasites are involved with HIV related diarrhoea by increasing the sample size.

For the present study, a small sample size was taken because of the technical reason(s) and financial constrains. One of the important limiting factors, for adopting a small sample size was lack of adequate fund as some lump sum amount had to be paid as monetary assistance to the HIV/AIDS patients towards conveyance for bringing the samples to the laboratory/ hospital.

Table 3.1 Seasonal prevalence of intestinal parasites associated with *ART naive* patients of Imphal District (January - December 2014)

Total no. of individual(s) examined: 288 Total no. of positive individual(s): 89

Month (s) / Parasite (s)	Sex	Jan	Feb	Mar	Apr	May	Jun	Jul	Aug	Sep	Oct	Nov	Dec
Ascaris lumbricoides	M	1	0	0	0	0	1	0	0	0	0	1	0
	F	0	0	0	0	0	1	0	1	0	0	0	0
Trichuris trichiura	M	0	0	0	1	0	0	0	0	0	0	0	0
	F	1	0	0	1	0	1	0	0	0	0	0	0
Hookworm	M	0	0	2	0	0	1	0	0	0	1	1	0
	F	0	0	0	0	1	2	0	1	0	0	0	0
Enterobius vermicularis	M	1	0	0	0	0	0	0	0	0	0	0	0
	F	1	0	0	0	1	0	3	2	1	0	0	0
Strongyloides stercoralis	M	0	0	1	0	0	2	1	0	0	0	0	0
	F	1	0	0	0	0	0	2	0	2	0	1	0
A. lumbricoides + Hookworm	M	0	0	0	1	0	0	0	3	0	0	0	0
	F	0	0	0	2	0	0	0	0	0	0	0	0
Cryptosporidium sp.	M	0	3	0	0	0	1	7	1	0	1	0	0
	F	0	0	1	0	2	1	1	0	3	0	0	0
Entamoeba histolytica	M	0	2	1	3	0	0	2	1	1	2	1	0
	F	2	1	0	0	4	0	0	0	0	2	3	0

Table 3.2 Seasonal prevalence of intestinal parasites associated with *On ART* patients of Imphal district (January - December 2015)

Total no. of individual(s) examined: 288 Total no. of positive individual(s): 21

Month (s) / Parasite (s)	Sex	Jan	Feb	Mar	Apr	May	Jun	Jul	Aug	Sep	Oct	Nov	Dec
Cryptosporidium sp.	M	0	0	0	1	0	0	0	0	0	1	0	0
	F	0	0	0	0	0	0	1	0	0	0	0	0
Entamoeba histolytica	M	0	0	1	0	0	1	1	0	1	0	1	0
	F	0	0	0	0	1	0	1	1	0	0	0	0
Hookworm	M	0	0	0	0	0	0	0	1	0	0	0	2
	F	0	0	0	0	0	1	0	0	2	0	0	0
Giardia lamblia	M	0	0	0	1	0	0	1	0	0	0	0	0
	F	0	0	0	0	0	0	0	2	0	0	0	0

Table 3.3 Environmental factor (s) and prevalence of Amoebiasis

Month (s)	Environmental factor(s)			No. of infected patient (s)
	Temperature (°C)	Rainfall (mm)	Relative Humidity (%)	
Jan '14	24	0	41.7	2
Feb ' 14	23.8	1.1	46.1	3
Mar '14	28	0.9	43.5	1
Apr ' 14	30.5	1.6	53.3	3
May '14	30.1	8.9	64.4	4
Jun '14	31	12.8	73.1	0
Jul '14	32.8	2.7	68.3	2
Aug '14	32	8.5	72	1
Sep '14	30.6	3.6	68.5	1
Oct '14	29.2	0.9	63.5	4
Nov '14	28	0	53.9	4
Dec '14	23.4	0	56.3	0

Table 3.4 Environmental factor (s) and prevalence of Cryptosporidiosis

Month (s)	Environmental factor(s)			No. of infected patient (s)
	Temperature (°C)	Rainfall (mm)	Relative Humidity (%)	
Jan '14	24	0	41.7	0
Feb ' 14	23.8	1.1	46.1	3
Mar '14	28	0.9	43.5	1
Apr ' 14	30.5	1.6	53.3	0
May '14	30.1	8.9	64.4	2
Jun '14	31	12.8	73.1	2
Jul '14	32.8	2.7	68.3	8
Aug '14	32	8.5	72	1
Sep '14	30.6	3.6	68.5	3
Oct '14	29.2	0.9	63.5	1
Nov '14	28	0	53.9	0
Dec '14	23.4	0	56.3	0

Fig 3.1: Graphical presentation of intestinal parasitic infections in HIV infected *ART naive* patients of Imphal District (Jan to Dec 2014)

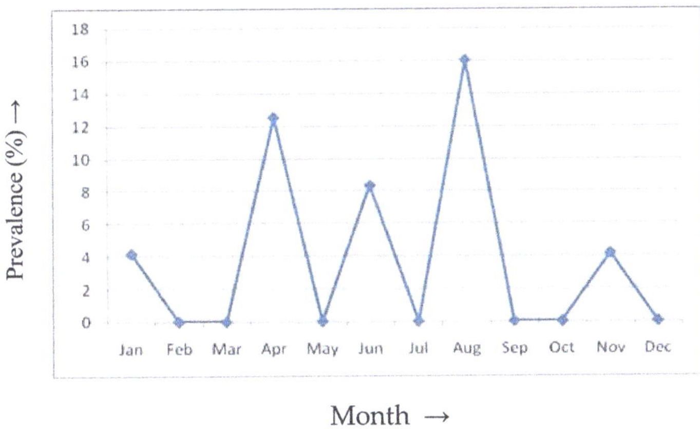

Fig. 3.1.1 Prevalence of Ascariasis in *ART naive* patients

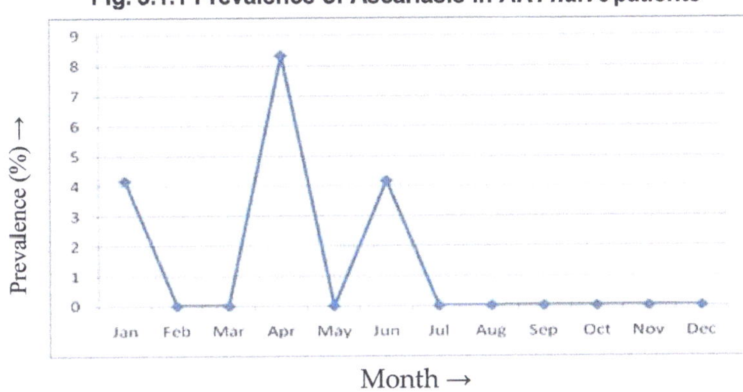

Fig. 3.1.2: Prevalence of Trichuriasis in *ART naive* patients

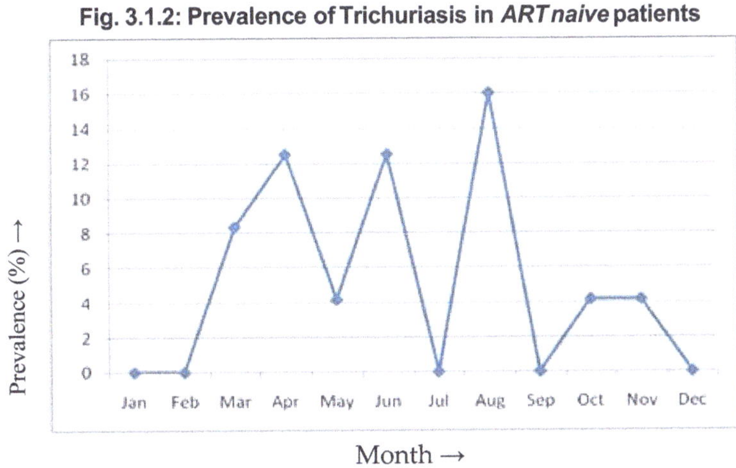

Fig. 3.1.3 Prevalence of Hookworm infection in *ART naive* patients

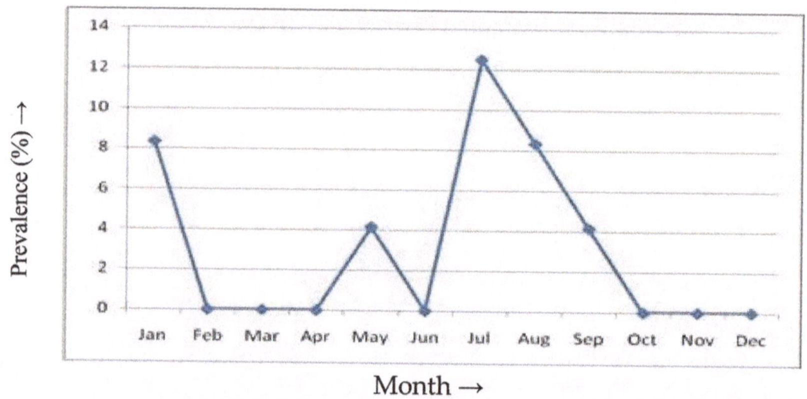

Fig. 3.1.4 Prevalence of Enterobiasis in *ARTnaive* HIV patients

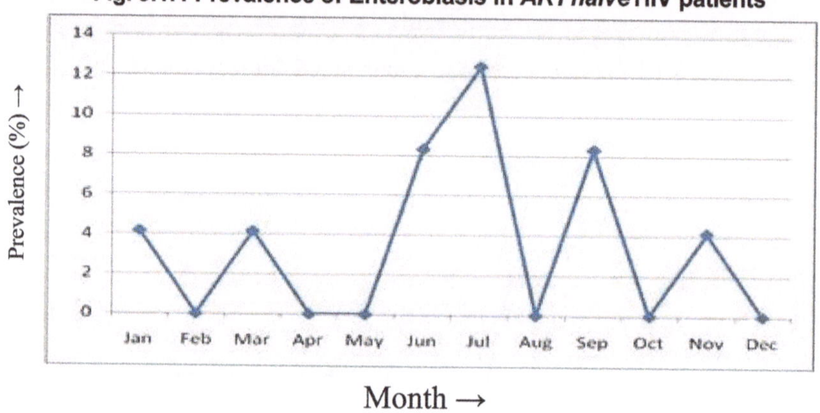

Fig. 3.1.5 Prevalence of Strongyloidiasis in *ARTnaive* patients

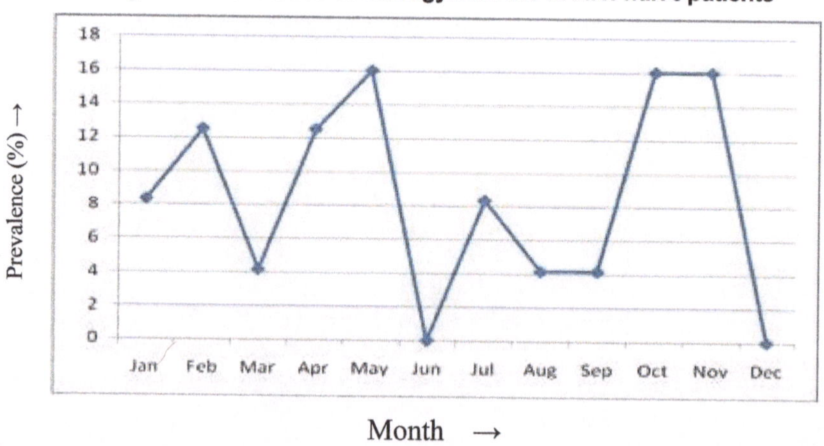

Fig. 3.1.6 Prevalence of Amoebiasis in ART naive HIV patients of Imphal District

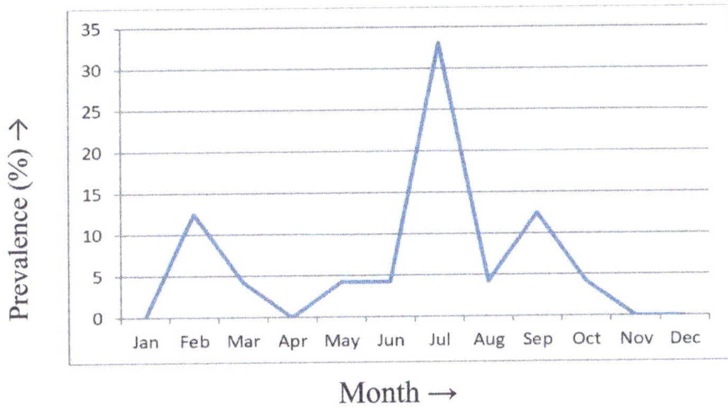

Fig. 3.1.7 Prevalence of Cryptosporidiosis in *ART naive* patients

Fig 3.2 Graphical presentation of intestinal parasitic infections in HIV infected *On ART* patients of Imphal District (Jan to Dec 2015)

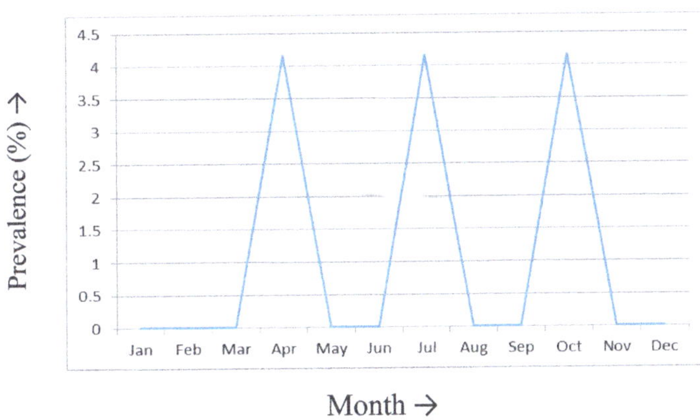

Fig. 3.2.1 Prevalence of Cryptosporidiosis in On ART patients

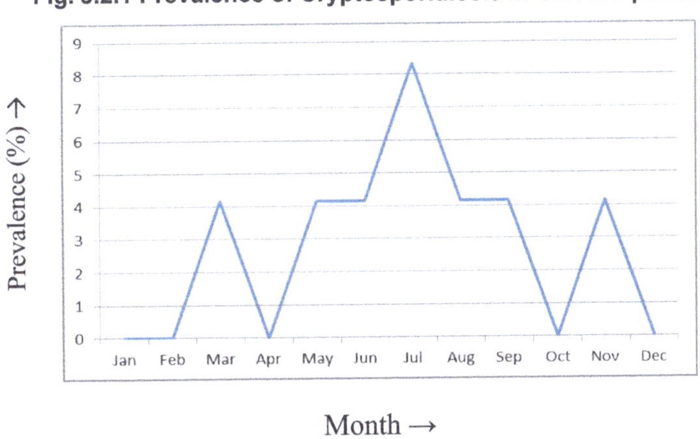

Fig. 3.2.2 Prevalence of Amoebiasis in *On ART* patients

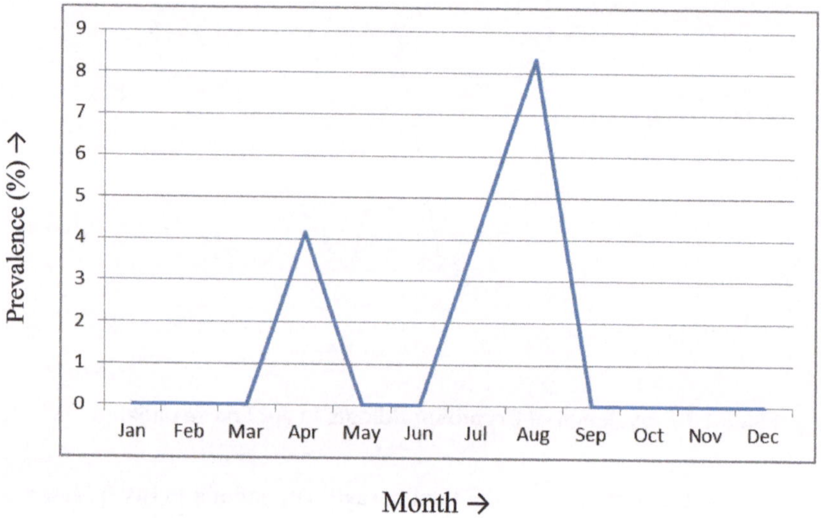

Fig. 3.2.3 Prevalence of Giardiasis in *On ART* patients

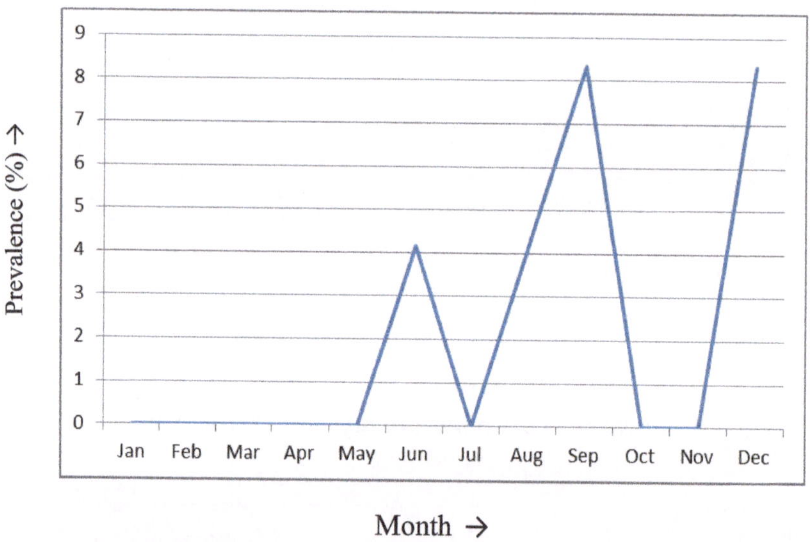

Fig. 3.2.4 Prevalence of Hookworm infection in *On ART* patients

7

Intestinal Parasitic Infection in Relation to CD_4 Count and HIV-1 RNA Plasma Viral Load in HIV Infected Patients

Introduction

Infection with HIV reduces the count of the Helper T cells (also known as CD_4 cells) and as their count decreases, the individual's immune system gets weakened/deteriorated and ultimately leads to an immuno-compromised/ immuno-suppressed state. The normal CD_4 count of an HIV seronegative healthy adult lies within the range of 500-1500 cells/µl of blood (Eligio-Garcia *et al.*, 2016). However, HIV seronegative healthy adult/individual(s) in Manipur have a CD_4 count within the range of 252 to 1449 cells/µl of blood (Lilavati *et al.*, 2016), revealing a lower CD_4 count much below the clinically significant level of 500 cells/µl. CD_4 counts are known to be influenced by race, physiological conditions and environmental factors. In a person with HIV infection, CD_4 count decrease on average by 20 - 30 cells/cu. mm of blood per year (Willy *et al.*, 2004).

As a result of the weak immune system or response, the patient becomes vulnerable to a number of infections including those caused by parasites. The number of Helper T cells (CD_4 cells) reflects the stage of infection in an HIV patient and this parameter is used to determine the immunity status (whether immunologically competent i.e. strong or not) of the individual/patient.

In Manipur, earlier workers had reported association of a number of enteric parasites like - *Cryptosporidium* sp., *Isospora belli, Entamoeba histolytica, Giardia lamblia, Cyclospora cayetanensis, Ascaris lumbricoides, Strongyloides stercoralis, Trichuris trichiura,* hookworm and *Enterobius vermicularis* etc. with PLHA without determining/monitoring their respective CD_4 cell counts and the HIV 1 RNA plasma viral load (Anand *et al.*, 1996; Anand *et al.*, 1998; Agarwal *et al.*, 1998; Singh *et al.*, 2004a & 2004b; Devi *et al.*,2010; Sherpa *et al.*, 2010; Sarkar *et al.*, 2012; Kamki *et al.*, 2015). These parasitic infections are often correlated with the CD_4 count of the individuals. Various workers have already done extensive work in this field

(Attili *et al.*, 2006; Dalvi *et al.*, 2006; Zope *et al.*, 2014; Eligio-Garcia *et al.*, 2016; Tay SCK *et al.*, 2017; Patel *et al.*, 2017). Similarly, these parasitic infections are also often correlated with the HIV-1 RNA plasma viral load of the patients (Wolday *et al.*, 2002; Endeshaw, 2005; Hosseinipour *et al.*, 2007; Kassu *et al.*, 2008; Walson *et al.*, 2008; Cardoso *et al.*, 2011; Ahmed *et al.*, 2013; Mulu *et al.*, 2013; Eligio-Garcia *et al.*, 2016). Moreover, there are reports that HIV patients having viral load values < 30,000 copies/ml are considered to have low probability to develop AIDS and death (Eligio-Garcia *et al.*, 2016).

However, in Manipur, no detailed and authentic work has been done till date towards establishing the relationship, if any, between i) enteric parasitic infection and CD_4 count and ii) enteric parasitic infection and HIV-1 RNA plasma viral load.

Therefore, with a view towards addressing this scientific discourse and with the aim of filling up this lacunae, in the context of the people living with HIV/AIDS in the state of Manipur, a study was carried out to unravel the relationship, if any, between the presence of enteric parasitic infection and that of the CD_4 count and HIV-1 RNA plasma viral load.

For this study, three stool samples (one fresh and the other two preserved in 4% $K_2Cr_2O_7$/PBS/4% formol saline) from 34 HIV positive antiretroviral treatment naive (*ART naive*) patients, aged between 19 to 50 years, who had visited the Viral Load Testing Lab and CD_4 count centre of the Department of Microbiology, RIMS hospital for determining/monitoring their CD_4 cells count and HIV-1 RNA plasma viral load status were collected. There were 13 males and 21 females. Of the 34 patients, 24 were diarrhoeal and 10 were non-diarrhoeal.

All the male patients were injecting drug users (IDU) and 7 females were commercial sex workers (CSW).

FACS count system and qRT PCR (Roche Cobas TaqMan 48 Analyzer) were employed for determining/monitoring the CD_4 count and HIV-1 RNA plasma viral load of the patient(s). The CD_4 count of the patients were categorized into three groups i.e. patients with CD_4 count < 200 cells/μl, within the range of 200 – 500 cells/μl and > 500 cells/μl (Devi, RH *et al.*, 2019) and HIV-1 RNA viral load of the patients were also categorized into 3 groups – Patients with low risk of HIV transmission [i.e. patients having HIV-1 RNA viral load value(s) < 10,000 copies/ml], Patients with medium risk of HIV transmission [i.e. patients having HIV-1 RNA viral load value(s) within the range of 10,000 – 49,999 copies/ml] and Patients with high risk of HIV transmission [i.e. patients having HIV-1 RNA viral load value(s) ≥ 50,000 copies/ml] (Murnane *et al.*, 2012) respectively.

In order to facilitate statistical analysis (χ^2 test), between the presence of parasitic infection and CD_4 count, the patients were categorized into two groups, i.e. group A, where the individuals were having normal CD_4 count value (i.e. within the range of 500 – 1500 cells/μl of blood) and group B, where the individuals had CD_4 count(s) beyond/outside the normal range (i.e. having CD_4 count either < 500 cells/μl or > 1500 cells/μl). Similarly, for studying the relationship, if any, between the presence of enteric parasitic infection and HIV-1 RNA viral load, patients were categorized into two groups, i.e. one group having HIV-1 RNA viral load value within the range of 1- 50,000 copies/ml and the other group having viral load value > 50,000 copies/ml.

Findings and Analysis

Of the 34 patients examined (Table 4.1), 19 patients (55.88%) were found positive for parasitic infection. Out of the 19 patients, there were 17 diarrhoeal and 2 non-diarrhoeal patients. During the present study, among the diarrhoeal patients, *Cryptosporidium* sp and *G. lamblia* were observed in 6 and 5 patients respectively while *A. lumbricoides*, hookworm and *S. stercoralis* were observed in 2 patients each. *E. histolytica* and *E. vermicularis* were observed in 1 patient each. Other than these pathogenic parasites, commensals like *Entamoeba coli, Endolimax nana* and *Chilomastix mesnili* were also observed among the patients.

The non-diarrhoeal patients were found to have harboured only *A. lumbricoides* and hookworm. None of the patients were found to be suffering from mixed infections.

Enteric parasites and CD_4 count

Table 4.2 shows the distribution of parasites among the different categories of CD_4 counts. The study revealed that cryptosporidiosis was observed in 6 patients. Out of which 5 patients had CD_4 count < 200 cells/μl while 1 patient had CD_4 count within the range of 200 – 500 cells/μl. Amoebiasis and giardiasis were observed in 1 and 5 patients respectively. The lone patient with amoebiasis had a CD_4 count within the range of 200-500 cells/μl. In case of giardiasis, a CD_4 count of < 200 cells/μl was observed in 3 patients and while a CD_4 count of > 500 cells/μl was observed in 1 patient, a CD_4 count within the range of 200-500 cells/μl was observed in the other patient.

Ascariasis was observed in 2 patients whose CD_4 counts were within the range of 200 – 500 cells/μl. Hookworm infection was observed in 2 patients, out of which 1 patient had a CD_4 count within the range of 200 – 500 cells/μl while the other patient had a CD_4 count > 500 cells/μl. In the present study, while enterobiasis was observed in a lone patient who had a CD_4 count > 500 cells/μl, strongyloidiasis was observed in 2 patients, out of which while 1 patient had a CD_4 count within the range of 200 - 500 cells/μl, the other had a CD_4 count > 500 cells/μl. In case of cryptosporidiosis, as 5 patients out of 6 had a CD_4 count < 200 cells/μl, it can be presumed that occurrence of this disease is higher in patients with low CD_4 count as far as the present study is concerned. However, the occurrence of other enteric helminthic infections seems to be more associated with patients having a CD_4 count ≥200 cells/μl.

Based on the findings of this study, it may also be inferred that while occurrence(s) of parasite(s), especially of G. *lamblia* and *Cryptosporidium* sp. were higher in patients who had CD_4 count < 200 cells/μl, occurrence rate of other parasite species was more in patients whose CD_4 count value lied within the range of 200-500 cells/μl.

The study shows that while maximum number of *Cryptosporidium* infected individual(s) were encountered in patients having low CD_4 count (< 200 cells/μl), patients suffering from giardiasis were observed to be independent of CD_4 count.

However, diseases like amoebiasis and other enteric helminthic infections were observed to have been associated with patients having a CD_4 count ≥200 cells/μl.

Statistical analysis revealed that presence of intestinal parasitic infection was independent of CD_4 count (χ^2 analysis, CV=0.005; TV= 3.841; df= 2; $P< 0.05$).

Enteric parasites and HIV-1 RNA viral load

Of the five patients infected with *G. lamblia*, while three patients had HIV-1 RNA viral load value(s) of 3,50,000, 2,74,000 and 1,21,000 copies/ml, all having HIV-1 RNA viral load value(s) ≥ 50,000 copies/ml; the other two patients had HIV-1 RNA value(s) of 6,990 and 34 copies/ml respectively.

The disease ascariasis was observed in two patients, out of which while one patient had an HIV-1 RNA viral load value of 2,98,000 copies/ml (i.e. this value falls under the category of ≥ 50,000 copies/ml), the other patient had a viral load value of 7,720 copies/ml (i.e. < 10,000 copies/ml).

Only two patients were found to have harboured *S. stercoralis.* Of the two patients, while one patient had an HIV-1 RNA viral load value of 56,900 copies/ml (i.e. ≥ 50,000 copies/ml) the other had an HIV-1 RNA viral load value of 4,230 copies/ml (i.e. < 10,000 copies/ml).

Of the six patients with cryptosporidial infection, while two patients had HIV-1 RNA viral load value(s) of 8,14,000 and 4,57,000 copies/ml (i.e. ≥ 50,000 copies/ml), viral load value(s) of 5,790 and 9,950 copies/ml (i.e. < 10,000 copies/ml) and 19,700 and 37,100 copies/ml (i.e. within the range of 10,000 – 49,999 copies/ml) were observed in each of the two patients respectively.

Of the two patients, who were diagnosed as suffering from hookworm infection, while one patient had an HIV-1 RNA viral load value of 1,370 copies/ml (i.e. < 10,000 copies/ml), an HIV-1 RNA viral load value of 29,200 copies/ml (i.e. within the range of 10,000 - 49,999 copies/ml) was recorded in the other patient. While a patient with medium risk of HIV transmission was harbouring *E. histolytica* (having an HIV-1 RNA viral load value of 12,500 copies/ml), another patient with low risk of HIV transmission was observed to have been infected with *E. vermicularis* (having an HIV-1 RNA viral load value of 8,700 copies/ml).

The study revealed that occurrence of *Cryptosporidium* was observed in all the three categories of patients, *i.e.* patients with HIV-1 RNA viral load value < 10,000 copies/ml (i.e. low risk of HIV transmission), within 10,000 -49,999 copies/ml (*i.e.* medium risk of HIV transmission) and ≥ 50,000 copies/ml (*i.e.* high risk of HIV transmission). Occurrence of *Ascaris lumbricoides* was observed in two patients, while one was having low, the other was having high risk of HIV transmission; like wise hookworm was also observed in two patients, of whom one belonged to low and the other belonged to medium risk of HIV transmission.

None of the patients with high risk of HIV transmission were found to have harboured these two parasites.

Strongyloides stercoralis and *Giardia lamblia* were found to have been associated with both the two categories of patients, i.e. patients having low and high risk of HIV transmission. *Enterobius vermicularis* was observed in only one patient who had low risk of HIV transmission. Similarly, *Entamoeba histolytica* was also observed in only one patient who had medium risk of HIV transmission.

On χ^2 analysis, it was observed that presence of intestinal parasitic infection was independent of HIV-1 RNA viral load value(s) [CV=1.145; TV=3.841; df = 2; $P < 0.05$; CV<TV]. Although a small sample size was taken for the present study, based on the present observation, it can be inferred that presence or absence of enteric parasitic infection(s) is not associated with variation(s) [either decrease or increase] in the HIV-1 RNA viral load in an HIV infected individual.

Table 4.1: Association of enteric parasites with CD4 count, HIV-1 RNA viral load and presence or absence of diarrhoea in *ARTnaive* patients (n=34)

Age/Sex	Diarrhoea	CD4 Count [Cells/µl]	Viral load [Copies/ml]	Parasite/Commensal Detected
48/M	+	343	6,990	*Giardia lamblia*
35/F	+	139	3,50,000	*Giardia lamblia*
26/M	+	301	7,720	*Ascaris lumbricoides*
50/F	+	170	5,790	*Cryptosporidium* sp
19/F	+	332	3,160	*Entamoeba coli*
48/F	+	589	32,700	*Entamoeba coli*
45/F	+	197	19,700	*Cryptosporidium* sp
47/M	+	326	54,000	*Endolimax nana*
40/F	+	525	41,900	*Entamoeba coli*
44/F	+	395	1,320	*Entamoeba coli*
40/F	+	200	56,900	*Strongyloides stercoralis*
36/F	+	666	1,370	Hookworm
30/F	+	54	8,14,000	*Cryptosporidium* sp
40/F	+	215	14,100	*Endolimax nana*

Age/Sex	Diarrhoea	CD_4 Count [Cells/µl]	Viral load [Copies/ml]	Parasite/Commensal Detected
23/M	+	776	34	*Giardia lamblia*
23/F	+	610	8,700	*Enterobius vermicularis*
23/F	+	447	12,500	*Entamoeba histolytica*
42/M	+	219	9,950	*Cryptosporidium* sp
26/M	+	109	4,57,000	*Cryptosporidium* sp
45/F	+	713	4,230	*Strongyloides stercoralis*
40/F	+	52	37,100	*Cryptosporidium* sp
26/F	+	34	2,74,000	*Giardia lamblia*
30/F	+	389	79,100	*Entamoeba coli*
40/M	-	58	1,62,000	*Endolimax nana*
37/M	-	648	9,220	*Entamoeba coli*
39/M	-	137	48,500	*Endolimax nana*
40/F	-	188	42,600	*Endolimax nana*
50/F	+	52	1,21,000	*Giardia lamblia*
45/M	-	09	5,080	*Endolimax nana*
26/F	-	263	23,400	*Endolimax nana*
23/F	-	370	6,370	*Entamoeba coli*
45/M	-	266	29,200	Hookworm
42/M	-	317	2,98,000	*Ascaris lumbricoides*
41/M	-	141	10,800	*Chilomastix mesnili*

Table 4.2: Distribution of enteric parasites in HIV positive *ART naive* patients having different categories of CD_4 count (n = 19)

Parasite(s) observed	Number of patient(s) in each category of CD_4 count(s) [Cells/µl]			
	< 200	200-500	> 500	Total no. of patient(s) positive for each species
G. lamblia	3	1	1	5
Cryptosporidium sp.	5	1	0	6
E. histolytica	0	1	0	1
A. lumbricoides	0	2	0	2
Hookworm	0	1	1	2
E. vermicularis	0	0	1	1
S. stercoralis	0	1	1	2
	08	07	04	19

Table 4.3: Distribution of enteric parasites in HIV positive *ARTnaive* patients having different categories of HIV 1 RNA viral load (n = 19)

Parasite(s) observed	Number of patient(s) in each category of HIV 1 RNA viral load [Copies/ml]			
	< 10,000	10,000 - 49,999	≥ 50,000	Total no. of patient(s) positive for each species
G. lamblia	2	0	3	5
Cryptosporidium sp.	2	2	2	6
E. histolytica	0	1	0	1
A. lumbricoides	1	0	1	2
Hookworm	1	1	0	2
E. vermicularis	1	0	0	1
S. stercoralis	1	0	1	2
	08	04	07	19

Discussion

Enteric parasites and CD_4 counts

In the present study, out of the 5 patients with giardiasis, while three patients had a CD_4 counts of < 200 cells/µl (the patients were having CD_4 counts of 34, 52 and 139 cells/µl), one patient had a CD_4 count within the range of 200 – 500 cells/µl (the patient was having a CD_4 count of 343 cells/µl) and the other patient had a CD_4 count > 500 cells/ µl (the patient had a CD_4count of 776 cells/µl) respectively. The present finding of giardiasis being observed in three patients having CD_4 counts of 34, 52 and 139 cells/µl is in agreement with the finding of Dalvi *et al.* (2006), who reported the occurrence of the disease in patients having a CD_4 count within the range 50-200 cells/µl. Moreover, the present observation of one patient having a CD_4 count of 343 cells/µl is in tally with the findings of Suryawanshi *et al.* (2012) and Surekha *et al.* (2016), who reported the observation of this disease in patients having CD_4 counts > 200 cells /µl and within the range of 200-500 cells / µl respectively.

Although in the present study, a patient with giardiasis was observed to have a CD_4 count of 776 cells/µl of blood, none of the above mentioned investigators reported a similar observation.

During this study, out of 6 patients with cryptosporidiosis, 5 patients had a CD_4 count < 200 cells/µl (the patients were having CD_4 counts of 52, 54, 109, 170, and 197 cells/µl) and 1 patient had a CD_4 count of > 200 cells/µl (i.e. 219 cells /µl). The present observation of two patients having CD_4counts of 52 and 54 cells/µl falls within the range of 32-106 cells/µl as reported by Attili *et al.* (2006).

Three cryptosporidiosis patients of the present investigation having CD_4 counts of 109, 170 and 197 cells/μl are also in agreement with the findings of Assefa *et al.* (2009), Venkatesh *et al.* (2012), Agarwal *et al.* (2015) and Surekha *et al.* (2016) who also reported the association of the disease with patients having CD_4 count < 200 cells/μl. The revelation of 1 patient of the present study being recorded with a CD_4 count of 219 cells/μl corroborates the observations of Assefa *et al.* (2009) and Surekha *et al.* (2016) who reported the occurrence of the disease in patients with CD_4 counts within the range of 200 - 349 cells/μl and > 200 cells/μl, i.e. 200 - 500 cells/μl.

The only patient diagnosed as suffering from amoebiasis was observed to have a CD_4 count of 447 cells/μl of blood. This finding is consistent with the findings of Venkatesh *et al.* (2012) and Surekha *et al.* (2016), who reported the occurrence of this disease in the HIV patients having CD_4 counts within the range of 200-500 cells/μl. However the present observation is not in tally with the findings of Attili *et al.* (2006) and Agarwal *et al.* (2015),who reported the occurrence of amoebiasis in patients having CD_4 counts within the range of 28 – 186 cells/μl and < 200 cells/μl.

The two patients with ascariasis were recorded to have CD_4 counts of 301 and 317 cells/μl of blood respectively. These values are well within the range of 200-500 cells/μl and this observation is in conformity with the finding of Venkatesh et *al.* (2012), who reported the association of this disease with patients having CD_4 counts within the range of 200-500 cells/μl. However, the present finding is contradictory with the finding of Attili *et al.* (2006) who reported the occurrence of helminth infection in those patients having CD_4 counts within the range of 125-155 cells/μl.

Hookworm infection was detected in two patients whose CD_4 counts were 266 and 666 cells/μl of blood respectively. This observation is in tune with the findings made by Suryawanshi *et al.* (2012) and Vankatesh *et al.* (2012) as these CD_4 count values are consistent with their observations. While the former reported the occurrence of this disease in patients having a CD_4 count of > 200 cells/μl, the latter reported the observation of this infection in patients with CD_4 count of > 500 cells/μl.

Strongyloidiasis was observed in two patients whose CD_4 counts were found to be 200 and 713 cells/μl of blood respectively. The present finding is contradictory with the observations of Suryawanshi *et al.* (2012) and Agarwal *et al.* (2015) who reported the occurrence of this disease in HIV patients having CD_4 count < 200 cells/μl. However, the present observation of a patient having a CD_4 count of 200 cells/μl fits well and is consistent with the findings of Assefa *et al.* (2009) and Venkatesh *et al.* (2012) who reported the presence of this disease in patients having CD_4 counts within the range of 200- 349 cells/μl and 200 - 500cells/μl. Moreover, the present observation of strongyloidiasis in a patient with a CD_4 count value of 713 cells/μl is in agreement with the finding of Assefa *et al.* (2009), who also reported the occurrence of this parasitic disease in HIV patients having CD_4 counts ≥500 cells/µl of blood.

In the present study, enterobiasis was observed in a patient whose CD_4 count value was found to be 610 cells/µl.

None of the currently referred /cited workers reported the observation of this disease among their studied population. During the present study, higher occurrence of cryptosporidiosis and giardiasis were observed in patients having a CD_4 count of < 200 cells/µl. The present finding of higher occurrence of enteric parasitosis in patients whose CD_4 count lies within the range of 200 – 500 cells/µl is contradictory with the finding of Sherpa *et al.* (2010), who reported intestinal parasitic infection to be more common in patients whose CD_4 count lies within the range of 100-200 cells/µl.

Enteric parasites and HIV-1 RNA Viral load

The present finding of cryptosporidiosis being prevalent in patients having HIV-1 RNA viral load value < 10,000 copies/ml is in conformity with the findings of Endeshaw (2005), who based on his study that was carried out in Ethiopia (South Africa) also reported the occurrence of this disease in HIV patients with HIV-1 RNA viral load value < 10,000 copies/ml. However, during the present study, although the disease was recorded in 33.3% of the studied population, Endeshaw (2005) observed the disease in only 10% of his studied population.

The present observation of HIV-1 RNA viral load value of 2,98,000 copies/ml in one of the two patients with ascariasis is in agreement with the findings of Walson *et al.* (2008) who reported a significant association between HIV-1 RNA level and ascariasis. During the study period, a number of HIV positive asymptomatic patients were observed to have harboured *A. lumbricoides*. In this regard, it may be mentioned that although treatment for these parasite positive patient(s) was done based on the laboratory findings/observations, by the Resident Medical Officer(s) of the drug de-addiction centre(s) to which the patient(s) were admitted /enrolled, no further follow up studies were done or carried out as the patients lacked participatory tendency. But, there are reports that eradication of *A. lumbricoides* from asymptomatic HIV-1 infected patients resulted in a significant elevation in the CD_4 counts and a trend towards a plasma HIV-1 RNA viral load decrease (Walson *et al.*, 2008).

Although there are reports that HIV-1 RNA plasma viral load was significantly higher in individuals with a helminthic infection (Mulu *et al.*, 2013), the present finding(s), although based on the observation(s) of a small sample size, do not corroborate the findings of Mulu *et al.* (2013).

Cardoso *et al.* (2011) based on a study in Sau Paulo, Brazil, reported the presence of *G. lamblia* in HIV-1 infected patients having a viral load value within the range of 10,000 – 1,00,000 copies/ml and this finding is contradictory with the present finding in which the presence of *G. lamblia* was observed in three patients who had an HIV-1 RNA viral load value > 1,00,000 copies/ml and in two patients who had HIV-1 RNA viral load value <10,000 copies/ml. The present observation of the presence of non-pathogenic amoeba – *Endolimax nana* in one patient who had an HIV-1 RNA viral load value > 1,00,000 copies/ml (the patient was having a viral load value of 1,62,000 copies/ml) is in conformity with the findings of Cardoso *et al.* (2011) who reported the occurrence of this non-pathogenic amoeba in patients who had appreciably high viral load (i.e. > 1,00,000 copies/ml). However, the present finding of *E. nana* in another six patients who had a viral load value < 10,000 copies/ml is contradictory with the findings of Cardoso *et al.* (2011), who reported the occurrence of *E. nana* in only those patients who had a superior viral load (i.e. > 1,00,000 copies/ml).

Although Cardoso *et al.* (2011) reported the detection of *Isospora belli* in 3 patients who had an HIV-1 RNA viral load value > 1,00,000 copies/ml, in the present study, none of the patients were found to have harboured this protozoan parasite.

The present finding, i.e. the presence of intestinal parasitic infection is independent of CD_4 count and HIV-1 RNA viral load is in close agreement with the findings of Kassu *et al.* (2008) and Eligio – Garcia *et al.* (2016), who also reported similar observations based on their studies in Ethiopia and Mexico respectively. However, the present observation is contradictory with the findings of Hosseinipour *et al.* (2007) who reported that among HIV infected patients helminth infections were associated with higher CD_4 count(s) but not with higher HIV-1 RNA levels. The present finding is also not in tally with the findings of Mulu *et al.* (2013) who reported helminths to be associated with patients having an increased HIV-1 RNA level.

Although Kassu *et al.* (2008) reported relatively higher viral load values in patients infected with *S. stercoralis* and hookworm, in the present study, patients harbouring *G. lamblia* and *Cryptosporidium* sp. were observed to have higher HIV-1 RNA viral load values.

References

Actor, I. , Mursunori, S. H. , Kulberg, M. , Buller, M. , Sher, A. and **Berzofsky, J. 1993**: Helminth infection results in decreased virus specific CD8+ cytotoxic T cell and Th-1 cytokine responses as well as delayed virus clearance. *Proc Natl Acad Sci, USA*, 90: 948-952.

Adamu, H. and **Petros, B. 2016**: Intestinal protozoan infections among HIV positive persons with and without antiretroviral treatment (ART) in selected ART Centers in Adama, Afar and Dire- Dawa, Ethiopia. *J Bacteriol Parasitol.* 7:5 (Suppl) http://dx.doi.org/10.4172/2155-9597 - C1.023.

Agarwal, A., Ningthouja, S., Sharma, D., Mohen, Y. and **Singh, Ng. B. 1998**: *Cryptosporidium* and HIV. *J Ind Med Asso.* 96(9): 276 – 277.

Aggarwal, A., Arora, U., Bajaj, R. and **Kumar, K. 2005**: Clinico-microbiological study in HIV seropositive patients. *J Ind Acad Clin Med.* 6(2): 142 - 145.

Agarwal, S.G., Powar, R. M., Tankhiwale, S. and **Rukadikar, A. 2015:** Study of opportunistic Infections in HIV-AIDS Patients and their Co –Relation with CD4+ Cell Count. *Int. J. Curr. Microbiol. App. Sci.* 4(6): 848-861.

Ahmad, H., Samantaray, J. C., Dar, L. Vajpayee, M. and **Sinha, S. 2013**: Treatment of parasitic infection in HIV-1 co-infected patients decrease HIV plasma load. *J Clin Exp Pathol.* DOI: 10.4172/2161-0681.

Akinbo, F.O., Okaka, C.E. and **Omoregie, R. 2010**: Prevalence of intestinal parasitic infections among HIV patients in Benin City, Nigeria. *Libyan J Med.* 5:10. 3402/ljm.v 5i0.5506 (Published online 2010 Oct 29 doi: 10.3402/ljm. v5i0.5506).

Amancio, FAM., Pascotto, VM., Souza, LR., Calvi, SA. and **Pereira, PCM., 2012:** Intestinal parasitic infections in HIV/AIDS patients: epidemiological, nutritional and immunological aspects. *J Venom Anim Toxins incl. Trop Dis* Vol. 18 No. 2 http:// dx. oi.org/10.1590 S1678-91992012000200013.

Anand, L., Brajachand, Ng. and **Dhanachand, Ch. 1996**: Cryptosporidiosis in HIV infection. *J Commun Dis.* 28(4): 241 - 244.

Anand, L., Dhanachand, Ch. and **Brajachand, Ng. 1998**: Prevalence and epidemiologic characteristics of opportunistic and non-opportunistic intestinal parasitic infections in HIV positive patients in Manipur. *J Commun Dis*.30 (1): 19 - 22.

Anand, L. 1999: Prevalence and epidemiology of human intestinal parasites in Manipur (Helminths & Protozoa) PhD Thesis, Manipur University (Unpublished)

Anon, 2001a: A Parasite Odyssey: workshop on HIV/AIDS, TB and co-infection with intestinal worms or helminths. Medical Research Council of South Africa News, October.Vol. 32: No.5.

Anon, 2001b: Encyclopaedic Reference of Parasitology, edited by Mehlhorn, H., Second edition, Springer, Germany. P- 462.

Anon, 2018: HIV Estimations 2017: Technical Report. New Delhi, NACO, Ministry of Health & Family Welfare, Government of India, National AIDS Control Organization & ICMR-National Institute of Medical Statistics.

Assefa, S., Erko, B., Medhin, G., Assefa, Z. and **Shimelis, T. 2009:** International parasitic infections in relation to HIV/AIDS status, diarrhoea and CD4 T- cell count. *BMC Infect Dis*. 9, 155: DOI: 10.1186/1471-2334-9-155.

Attili, S.V.S., Gulati, A.K., Singh, V.P., Varma, D.V., Rai, M. and **Shyam, S. 2006**: Diarrhoea, CD4 counts and enteric infections in a hospital- based cohort of HIV- infected patients around Varanasi, India. *BMC Infect Dis*. 6, 39: doi: 10.1186/1417-2334-6-39.

Ayyagari, A., Sharma, A. K., Prasad, K.N., Ghole, T.N., Kishore, J. and **Chaudhary, G. 1999**: Spectrum of opportunistic infections in Human Immunodeficiency Virus (H IV) infected cases in a tertiary care hospital. *Ind J Med Microbiol*. 17(2): 78 - 80.

Bachur, T.P.R., Vale, J.M., Coelho, I.C.B., Sales de Queiroz, T.R.B. and **Chaves, C. 2008**: Enteric parasitic infections in HIV/AIDS patients before and after the highly active antiretroviral therapy. *Braz J Infect Dis*. 12 (2): 115 – 122. http://dx.doi.org/10.1590/S1413-86702008000200004.

Baum, M. K., Phillips J. C., Sales, S., Daniel, V., Yang, Z., Yang A. and **Canpa, A. 2003**: Eosinophilia is associated with HIV disease progression. Keystone Symposia in Alberta, Canada, March 19- April 4, Abstract- 405.

Beaglehole, R., Bonita, R. and **Kjellstrom 1994**: Basic Epidemiology (Authorised Reprint) Published by WHO, reprinted in India by Orient Longman Ltd.

Beaver, P.C. 1975: Biology of soil-transmitted helminths: the massive infection. Health Laboratory Science, 12, 116 – 125.

Belding, D. 1965: Text book of Parasitology. Meredeth, New York, P 397 – 398

Bentwich, Z., Weisman. Z., Moroz, C., Bar- Yehud, S. and **Kalinkovich, A. 1996**: Immune dysregulation in Ethiopian immigrants in Israel: relevance to helminth infection. *Clin Exper Immunol*. 103: 239-243.

Bentwiz, Z. 1999: Can eradication of helminthic infections change the face of AIDS and tuberculosis. *Immunology Today*. 20: 485-487.

Blessman, J. and **Tannide, E. 2002**: Treatment of asymptomatic intestinal *Entamoeba histolytica* infection. *N Eng J Med* 347: 1384 - 1385

Borkow, G. and **Bentwich, Z. 2000**: Eradication of helminthic infections may be essential for successful vaccination against HIV and tuberculosis. *Bulletin of World Health Organization*. 78 (11): 1368-1369.

Borkow, G., Weisman, Z., Leng, Q., Stein, M., Kalinkovich, A., Wolday, D. and **Bentwich, Z. 2001**: Helminths, human immunodeficiency virus and tuberculosis. *Scand J Infect Dis*. 33: 568-571.

Brown, H.W. 1927: Studies on the rate of development and viability of the eggs of *Ascaris lumbricoides* and *Trichuris trichiura* under field conditions. *J Parasitol*, 14, 1 – 15.

Brown, M., Reed, S., Levy, J. A., Busch, M. and **McKerrow, J. H. 1991**: Detection of HIV-1 in *Entamoeba histolytica* without evidence of transmission to human cells. *AIDS* 5 (1): 93-96.

Brown, M., Kizza, M., Watera, Ch., Quigley, M.A., Rowland, S., Hughes, P., Whitworth, J. A. G. and **Elliott, A. M. 2004**: Helminth infection is not associated with faster progression of HIV disease in co infected adults in Uganda. *J Infect Dis*. 190: 1869-1879.

Bu Figueroa, E., Fernandez. J. and **Alvarado, T. 1992**: Caracteristicas epidemiologicas y clinicas de los 100 primeros casos de SIDA en Honduras. *Med Clin*. 1: 9-13.

Bundy, D. A. P. Sher, A. and **Michael, E. 2000**: Good worms or Bad worms, do worm infections affect the epidemiological pattern of other diseases? *Parasitol Today*. 16: 273-274.

Burchard, G. D., Hufert, F. T. and **Mirelman, D. 1991**: Characterization of 20 *Entamoeba histolytica* strains isolated from patients with HIV infection. *Infection*. 19 (3): 164-169.

Bushen, O. Y., Davenport, J. A., Lima, A. B., Piscitelli, S. C., Uzgiris, A. J., Silva, T. M. J., Leite, R., Kosek, M., Dillingham, R. A., Girao, A., Lima, A. A. M. and **Guerrant, R. L. 2004**: Diarrhoea and reduced levels of antiretroviral drugs: improvement with glutamine or alanayl-glutamine in a randomized controlled trial in northeast Brazil. *Clin Infect Dis*. 38 (12): 1764-1770.

Cardoso, L.V., Galisteu, K. J., Junior, A. S., Chahla, L. A. O. A., Canille, R. M.

S., Beleoto, M. V. T., Franco, C., Maia, I. L., Rossit, A. R. B. and **Machado, R. L. D. 2011**: Enteric parasites in HIV-1/AIDS – infected patients from a Northwestern Sao Paulo reference unit in the highly active antiretroviral therapy era. *Revista da Sociedade Brasileira de Medicina Tropical* 44(6): 665 - 669.

Carvalho, E .M. and **DA Fonseca Porto, A. 2004**: Epidemiological and clinical interaction between HTLV-1 and *Strongyloides stercoralis. Parasite Immunology.* 26: 487-497.

Castello-Branco, L. R. R., Lewis, D. J. M., Ortigao-de–Sampaio, M. B. and **Griffin, G. E. 1996**: Gastrointestinal immune response in HIV infected subjects. *Mem Inst Oswaldo Cruz.* 91: 263-266.

Chandora, A., Khatri, P.K., Meena, S., Bora, A., Rathore, L., Maurya, V. and **Sirvi, K. 2015**: Co-infection with *Cryptosporidium, Isospora* and *Giardia lamblia* in a patient living with HIV and AIDS – a Case Report. *Sch J App Med Sci.* 3(5C): 1975 - 1977.

Chatterjee, K. D. 2011: Parasitology (Protozoology and Helminthology) in relation to Clinical Medicine, 13th Edition, Chatterjee Medical Publishers, Calcutta, India, Pp 208-212.

Chavan, N.S. and **Chavan, S.N. 2014**: Intestinal parasitic infections in HIV infected patients. *Int J Curr Microbiol App Sci* 3(2): 265 - 270.

Cheesbrough, M. 2002: District Laboratory Practice in Tropical Countries, Part 1, Cambridge Low Price Editions, Cambridge University Press.

Chhin, S., Harwell, J.I., Bell, J.D., Rozycki, G., Ellman, T., Barnett, J. M., Ward, H., Reinert, S. E. and **Pugatch, D. 2006**: Etiology of chronic Diarrhoea in Antiretroviral naive patients with HIV infection admitted to Norodom Sihanouk hospital, Phnom Penh, Cambodia. *Clin Infect Dis* 43: 925 - 932.

Cimerman, S., Cimerman, B. and **Lewis, D.B. 1999**: Prevalence of intestinal parasitic infection in patients with Acquired Immunodeficiency Syndrome in Brazil. *Int J Infect Dis* 3:203 - 206.

Clasen, T., Schmidt, W.P., Rabie, T., Cairncross, S. and **Luby. 2007**: Interventions to improve water quality for preventing diarrhoea: systematic review and meta-analysis. *Brit Med J* 334 (7597): 782.

Cotte, L., Rabodonirina, M., Piens, M. A., Perreard, M., Mojon, M. and **Trepo, C. 1993**: Prevalence of internal protozoans in French patients infected with HIV. *J Acquir Immune Defic Syndr* 6: 1424-1429.

Connolly, K.J. and **Kvalsvig, J. D. 1992**: Infection, nutrition and cognitive performance in children. *Parasitol Today.* 104: S187-S200.

Cooper. 2001: A Parasite Odyssey: workshop on HIV/AIDS, TB and co-infection with intestinal worms or helminthes. Medical Research Council of South Africa News, October, Vol. 32: No.5.

Crompton, D.W.T. and **Pawlowski, Z.S. 1985**: Life history and development of *Ascaris lumbricoides* and the persistence of human ascariasis, In *Ascariasis and its public health significance* (editors: Crompton D.W.T, Nesheim M.C. Pawlowski, Z.S), Taylor and Francis, New York, London, Philadelphia. Pp 9-23.

Croxson, S., Mildvan, D., Mathews, H. and Poiesz, B.J. 1988: Entamoeba histolytica antigen specific induction of Human Immunodeficiency Virus replication. *J Clin Microbiol.* 26(7):1304 - 1308.

Curtis, V. and **Cairncross, S. 2003**: Effect of washing hands with soap on diarrhoea risk in the community: a systematic review. *Lancet infects Dis.* 3(5): 275-281.

Dalvi, S., Koticha, A., Mehta, P., Kedare, K. and **Nataraj, G. 2006**: Cyclosporiasis in HIV infected individuals: Two case reports. *Bom Hosp J* 48 (4): 652 - 654.

Darji, S.M., Pethani, J.D., Shah, P.D. and **Kadam, M.T. 2013**: Study of intestinal parasitic infection in HIV infected patients. *GCSMC J Med Sci* II (II): 24 - 26.

Devi, P. P., H., Rebachandra, Brajachand, S. Ng. and **Nabakumar, S.**

Th. 2010: *Strongyloides stercoralis* infection in an HIV positive patient – A case report from RIMS, Imphal, Manipur. *J Commun Dis.* 42 (3): 231-234.

Devi, R.H., Th, N.S., Singh, A.L. and Singh, R.K.G. 2019: Enteric parasitosis and its correlation with CD4 count in human immunodeficiency virus infected patients. *Int J Res Med Sci* 7(7) 2690 - 2695.

Dhanachand, Ch. and **Anand, L. 2003:** Helminthic infections in HIV/AIDS patients, In Helminthology in India (ISBN-81-7089-293-7); Edited by Prof. M.L. Sood, 2003 (International Book Distributors, Dehradun, India).

Didier, E.S., Orenstein, J.M., Aldras, A., Bertucci, D., Rogers, L.B. and **Janney, F.A. 1995:** Comparison of three staining methods for detecting Microsporidia in fluids. *J Clin Microbiol.* 33: 3138 – 3145.

Eligio - Garcia, L., Cano - Estrada, A., Cruz, C. and **Jimenez – Cardoso, E. 2016**: Association of viral load and CD4+ count with infection of intestinal emerging parasites in HIV patients. *J AIDS Clin Res.* 7 (12) DOI: 10.4172/2155 - 6113.1000644.

Endeshaw, T. 2005: Opportunistic and other intestinal parasites among HIV/ AIDS patients in Ethiopia. PhD Dissertation, Addis Ababa

University, Ethiopia, February, 2005.

Escobedo, A.A. and **Nunez, F. A. 1999:** Prevalence of intestinal parasites in Cuban acquired immune deficiency syndrome (AIDS) patients. *Acta Tropica.* 72:125 - 130.

Feitosa, G., Banbeira, A.C., Sampaio, D.P., Badaro, R. and **Brites, C. 2001**: High prevalence of giardiasis and stongyloidiasis among HIV- infected patients in Bahia, *Braz J Infect Dis* 5(6) Salvador ON- line version ISSN 1678-4391.

Fewtrell, L., Kaufmall, R. B., Kay, D., Enanoria, W., Haller, L. and **Colford Jr, J. M. 2005**: Water, sanitation and hygiene interventions to reduce diarrhoea in less developed countries: a systematic review and meta-analysis. *Lancet Infect Dis.* 5 (1): 42-52.

Fincham. 2001: Helminth, HIV/AIDS and Tuberculosis. AIDS Bulletin. Dec 2001, Vol.10: No.3.

Fontanet, A.L., Sahlu,T., Rinke, W.T. and **Coutinho, R.A. 2000**: Epidemiology of infection with Intestinal parasites and human immunodeficiency virus (HIV) among sugar –estate in Ethiopia. *Ann Trop Med Parasitol.* 94 (3): 269-78.

Goon, A.M., Gupta, M.K. and **Dasgupta, B. 1987**: Fundamentals of Statistics, Vol. 1, The World Press Private Ltd, Calcutta.

Gray, 2001: A Parasite Odyssey: workshop on HIV/AIDS, TB and co infection with intestinal worms or helminths. Medical Research Council of South Africa News, October. Vol. 32: No.5.

Guerrant, R.L., Huges, J.M., Lima, N.L. and **Crane, J. 1990**: Diarrhoea in developed and developing countries: magnitude, special settings, and etiologies. *Rev Infect Dis.* 12(suppl): S 41-50.

Hira, S.K., Shroff, H.J., Lanjewar, D.N., Dholkia, Y.N., Bhatia, V.P. and **Dupont, H.L. 2003**: The natural history of Human immunodeficiency virus infection among adults in Mumbai. *Natl Med J India.* 16:126-131.

Hosseinipour, M.C., Napravnik, S., Joaki, G., Gama, S., Mbeye, N., Banda, B., Martinson, F., Hoffman, I. and **Cohen, M.S. 2007**: HIV and parasitic infection and the effect of treatment among adult outpatients in Malawi. *J Infect Dis* 195(9): 1278 - 1282.

Howe, G.M. 1977: A world geography of Human Diseases. Academic Press, New York.

Hunter, G.W., Swartzwelder, J.C. and Clyde, D.F. 1976: Tropical Medicine 5th Edition, Philadelphia, WB Saunders Pp 465 -471.

Hunter, G., Bagshawe, A.F., Baboo, K.S., Luke, R. and **Provice, P. 1992**: Intestinal parasites in Zambian patients with AIDS. *Trans R Soc Trop Med Hyg* 86: 543 - 545.

Hunter, P.R. and **Nichols, G. 2002**: Epidemiology and clinical features of cryptosporidium infection in immuno-compromised patients. *Clin Microbiol Rev.* 1(10): 145-154.

Ichhpujani, R. L. and **Bhatia, R. 1999**: Medical Parasitology, Second Edition, Jaypee Brothers, New Delhi.

Inungu, J. N., Morse, A.A. and **Gordon, C. 2000**: Risk factors, seasonality and trends of cryptosporidiosis among patients infected with Human immunodeficiency virus *Am J Trop Med Hyg.* 62(3): 384-387.

John, D. T. and **Petri Jr., W. A. 2009**: Examination of stool specimens (Chapter 14), In Markell and Voge's Medical Parasitology, 9th Edition, Elsevier. P 407 – 408.

Kadappu, K.K., Nagaraja, M.V., Rao, P.V. and **Sastry, B.A. 2002**: Azithromycin as treatment for cryptosporidiosis in human immunodeficiency virus disease *J Postgrad Med.* 48:179-181.

Kalinkovich, A., Weisman, Z., Greenberg, Z., Nahmias, J., Etian, S., Stein, M. and **Bentwich, R. 1998**: Decreased CD4 and decreased CD8 counts with T-cell activation is associated with chronic helminth infection. *Clin Exp Immunol.* 114: 414-421.

Kaminskyl, R. G., Soto, R. J., Campa, A. and **Baum, M. K. 2004**: Intestinal parasitic infection and eosinophilia in a human immune deficiency virus positive population in Honduras. *Mem Inst Oswaldo Cruz* 99 (7): 773 - 778.

Kamki, Y., Singh, R.H., Singh, N. T., Lungram, P. and **Singh, B. N. 2015**: Intestinal protozoal and helminthic infections in immuno-compromised patients attending RIMS hospital, Imphal. *J Med Soc* 29(2): 74-78

Kassu, A., Fujino, M., Nishizawa, M., Mengistu, G., Diro, E., Ayele, B., Ketema, D., Moges, F., Mulu, A., Yismaw, G., Huruy, K., Abate, E., Getachew, A., Tiruneh, M., Wondmikun, Y., Sugiura, W. and **Ota, F. 2008**: Levels of serum HIV-1 RNA viral load in tuberculosis patients with or without intestinal parasites during treatment of tuberculosis in Gondar, Ethiopia. *Ethiop J Health Biomed Sci* 1(1): 3 - 10.

Kumar, S.S., Ananthan, S. and **Lakshmi, P. 2002**: Intestinal parasitic infection in HIV infected patients with diarrhoea in Chennai. *Ind J Med Microbiol* 20 (2):88 - 91.

Kreier, J.P. 1993: Parasitic Protozoa, Vol. 6, Second Edition, Academic Press. Pp. 192-193.

Lilavati, N., Roy, A., Marak, E., Laldnmawii, G., Singh, H. R. and **Devi Kh. S. 2016:** Enumeration of CD_4+ T lymphocytes count among healthy HIV seronegative individuals & people living with HIV in Manipur. *Int J Biomed Resh* 7(7): 430 -434.

Lule, J. R., Mermin, J., Ekwaru, J.P., Malamba, S., Downing, R., Ransom, R., Nakanjako, D., Wafula, W., Hughes, P., Bunnell, R., Kaharuza, F., Coutinho, A., Kigozi, A. and **Quick, R. 2005**: Effect of home based water chlorination and safe storage on diarrhea among persons with human immunodeficiency virus in Uganda. *Am J Trop Med Hyg.* 73 (5): 926-933.

May, J.M. 1958: Studies in Disease Ecology, MD publication, New York.

Mazumder, P.P., Bharati, P., Banerjee, D. and Basu, A. 1984: Dietary status in Chapota, Inter and Intra economic group variations. ISI Tech Report No. Anthrop/2/84.

Mendez, O.C., Szmulewicz, G. and **Gatta, C. 1994**: Comparison of intestinal parasite infestation indexes among HIV positive and negative population. *Medicina*. 54 (4): 307-10.

Misra, S.N., Sengupta, D. and **Satpathy, S.K. 1998**: AIDS in India: Recent trends in opportunistic infection. *South East Asian J Trop Med Publ Hlth*. 29: 373-376.

Missaye, A., Dagnew, M. and **Alemu, A. 2013**: Prevalence of intestinal parasites and associated risk factors among HIV/AIDS patients with Pre- ART and On- ART attending dessie hospital ART clinic, Northeast Ethiopia. *AIDS Resh Ther*. 10:7. DOI: 10.1186/1742-6405-10-7.

Montresor, A, Crompton, DWT, Hall, A., Bundy, DAP and **Savioli, L. 1998**: Guidelines for the evaluation of soil transmitted helminthiasis and schistosomiasis at community level. HO/CTD/SIP/98.1

Mukhopadhya, A., Ramakrishna, B. S., Gangadeep, K., Pulimood, A.B., Mathan, M.M. and Zachariah, A. 1999: Enteric pathogens in Southern Indian HIV infected patients with and without diarrhoea, *Ind J Med Resh*. 109, 85-89.

Mulu, A., Maier, M. and **Liebert, U.G. 2013**: Deworming of intestinal helminths reduces HIV-1 subtype C viremia in chronically co-infected individuals. *Int J Infect Dis*. 17(10): e897- e901.

Murnane, P.M., Hughes, J.P., Celum, C., Lingappa, J.R., Mugo, N., Farquhar, C., Kiarie, J., Wald, A. and Baeten, J. M. 2012: Using plasma viral load to guide antiretroviral therapy initiation to prevent HIV-1 transmission. PLOS ONE. 7(11) e51192 DOI: 10.1371/journal.pone.0051192.

Mwinzi, 2001: A Parasite Odyssey: workshop on HIV/AIDS, TB and co infection with intestinal worms or helminths. Medical Research Council of South Africa News, October. Vol. 32: No.5.

Nath, R., Saikia, L., Sen, S. S. and Borthakur, A. K. 2006: Clinical profile of HIV/ AIDS in Assam. Poster presentation (PM - 10), International Conference on Opportunistic pathogens in AIDS (ICOPA), New Delhi, 27 – 29 March, 2006.

Navin, T.R., Weber, R., Vugia, D.J., Rimlan, D., Roberts, J.M., Addis, D.G., Visvesvara, G.S., Wahlquist, S.P., Hogan, S.E., Gallager, L.E., Juranek, D.D., Schartz, D.A., Wilcox, C.M., Stewart, J.M., Thompson, S.E. III and Bryan, R.T. 1998: Declining CD4 T – lymphocyte counts are associated with increased risk of enteric parasitosis and chronic diarrhoea: Results of a 3 year longitudinal study. *J AIDS Hum Retrovirol*. 20, 154 – 159.

Nennis, N. 1992: Opportunistic infections in AIDS, Diagnostic Manual Workshop Manual, Department of Microbiology, St. Vincent Hospital, Sydney, Australia.

Niehaus, M.D., Moore, S.R., Patrick, P.D., Derr, L. L., Lorntz, B., Lima, A. A. and **Guerrant, R. L. 2002**: Early childhood diarrhoea is associated with diminished cognitive function 4 to 7 years later in children in a northeast Brazilian shantytown. *Trop Med Hyg*. 66 (5): 590-593.

Nokes, C. and **Bundy, DAP. 1993**: Compliance and absenteeism in school children implications for helminth control. *Trans R Soc Trop Med Hyg*. 87:148-152.

Oldfield, E.C. 2002: Evaluation of chronic diarrhoea in patients with human immunodeficiency virus infection. *Rev Gastroenterol Disord*. 2, 176 - 188.

Patel, S.D., Javadekar, T.B. and **Kinariwala, D.M. 2015**: Enteric opportunistic parasitic infections in HIV seropositive patients at tertiary care teaching hospital. *Natl J Med Resh* 5(3): 190 – 193.

Patel, M., Patel, R. and **Paliwal, M. 2017**: Intestinal parasitic infections in HIV -1 sero-positive individuals and its correlation with CD4 cell count in a tertiary care teaching hospital, Gujarat. *Intl J Biomed Adv Resh* 08 (04):174 – 178 (DOI: https://dx.doi.org/10.7439/ijbar).

Pozio, E. and Morales, M.A.G. 2005: The impact of HIV – protease inhibitors on opportunistic parasites. *Trends in Parasitology* 21(2) 58 – 63.

Prasad, S. 1997: Fundamentals of Biostatistics (Biometry), Emkay Publications, B – 19, East Krishna Nagar, Delhi – 110 051.

Ram Mohan, M., Nagamani, K. and **Saxena, N.K. 2013**: Enteric parasites in HIV/ AIDS patients: Study of the prevalence and risk factors. *Intl J Biomed Resh.* DOI:10.7439/ijbr CODEN: IJBRFA.

Ranjana, H. and **Singh, R.K.G. 2015**: Gastrointestinal parasites associated with HIV infected antiretroviral naive patients. *J Interacad* 19 (2), 216 - 223.

Ranjana, H., Singh, R.K.G., Singh, L.A. and **Singh, Ng. B. 2015**: *Strongyloides stercoralis* and hookworm co-infection in an HIV positive patient. *J Interacad* 19 (3): 403 - 409.

Ranjana, H., Anand, L. and **Singh, R.K.G. 2016**: *Ascaris lumbricoides* and *Strongyloides stercoralis* associated diarrhoea in an immunocompromised patient. *IOSR J Pharm Biol Sc.* 11 (5): Ver. IV (Sept. – Oct. 2016) 29 – 32.

Sarkar, A., Singh, H.R., Pukhrambam, P.D. and **Singh, Ng.B. 2012**: Opportunistic *Strongyloides stercoralis* infection in an immuno-compromised patient. *Ind Med Gazt.* Dec 497-500.

Savioli, L., Stansfield, S., Bundy, DAP, Mitchell, A., Bhatia, R., Engels, D., Montresor, A., Neira, M. and **Shein, A.M. 2002**: Schistosomiasis and soil transmitted helminhic infestation: foregoing control effects. *Trans R Soc Trop Med Hyg* 96: 577-579.

Sherpa, U., Devi, K. Mamta, Bhagyabati, S., Devi, Kh. Sulochana and **Singh, Ng.B. 2010**: Opportunistic intestinal parasitic infections in individuals with HIV/AIDS in RIMS hospital. *J Med Soc.* 24 (1): 8-11.

Singh, L.A., Das, S.C. and **Baruah, I. 2004a**: Enteric parasites in patients with HIV infection. *J Parasit Appl Anim Biol.* 13(1&2): 55-64.

Singh, L.A., Chinglensana, L., Singh, Ng. B., Singh H.L. and **Singh, Y.I. 2004b**: Helminthiasis in HIV infection: A brief report from Manipur (India). *J Commun Dis* 36(4): 293 -295.

Smith, H. V. 2002: Intestinal Protozoa, In Medical Parasitology, A Practical Approach, Edited by Gillespie, S.H. & Hawkey, P. M., Oxford University Press, Repinted. 2002, Pp 79-117.

Soave, R. 1996: Cyclospora: An overview, *Clin Infect Dis*, 23,429-437.

Sorvillo, F.J., Lieb, L.E., Siedel, J., Kerndt, P., Turner, J. and **Ash, L.R. 1995**: Epidemiology of isosporiasis among persons with acquired immunodeficiency syndrome in Los Angeles County. *Am J Trop Med Hyg*. 53: 656-659.

Stephenson, L.S., Lantham, M.C., Kinoti, S.N., Kurz, K.M. and **Brigham, H. 1990**: Improvement of physical fitness of Kenyan school boys infected with hookworm, *Trichuris trichiura* and *Ascaris lumbricoides* following a single dose of albendazole. *Trans R Soc Trop Med Hyg*. 84: 277-282.

Stephenson, L.S. 1994: Helminth infections: a major factor in malnutrition.World Health Forum 15: 169-172.

Storey, G.W. and **Phillips, R.A. 1985:** The survival of parasite eggs throughout the soil profile. *Parasitol* 91, 585 – 590.

Suryawanshi, M., Kalshetti, V., Telele, K., Wadile, Haswani, N. and **Ahire, K. 2012:** Intestinal Parasitic infections and the CD4 counts in HIV Seropositive Individuals in the Dhule District in Maharashtra, India. *J Clin Diagn Resh* 6 (7):1207-1209.

Surekha, Y. A., Shilpa, H. S., Jeer, M. and Krishna, S. 2016: Opportunistic intestinal parasites in HIV infected individuals and its correlation with the CD4 counts. *Int J Curr Microbiol App Sci* 5(2): 279-283.

Taklemarian, Z., Abate, D., Mitiku, H. and Dessie, Y. 2013: Prevalence of intestinal parasitic infection among HIV positive persons who are naïve and on Antiretroviral treatment in Hiwot Fana Specialized University Hospital, Eastern Ethiopia. ISRN AIDS http://dx.doi.org/10.1155/2013/324329.

Tay, S.C.K., Aryee, E.N.O. and Badu, K. 2017: Intestinal parasitemia and HIV/ AIDS co-infections at varying $CD4^+$ T-cell levels. *HIV/AIDS Res Treat Open J* 4(1): 40-48.

Venkatesh, N. R., Prakash H. R., PM, U., Vijayanath,V., Shreeharsha, V and **Chandak, V. K . 2012**: Opportunistic Parasitic Infections in HIV/AIDS Patients Presenting with Diarrhoea and their Correlation with CD_4+ T- Lymphocytes counts. *Int J Pharm Bio Sci* 2(4): 293-299.

Walson, J. L., Otieno, P. A., Mbuchi, M., Richardson, B. A., Lohman-payne, B., Macharia, S. W., Overbaugh, J., Berkley, J. S., Sanders, E. J., Chung, M. H.

and **John-Stewart, G. C. 2008**: Albendazole treatment among adults with HIV-1 and helminth co-infection: a randomized double blind placebo trial. *AIDS* 22: 1601-1609.

Weber, R., Lendergerber, B., Zbinden, R., Altwegg, M., Pfyffer, G. E., Spycher, M. A., Briner, J., Kaiser, L., Opravil, M., Meyenberger, C. and Flepp, M. 1999: Enteric infections and diarrhoea in human immunodeficiency virus infected persons *Arch Intern Med* 159:1473-1480. doi: 10.1001/ archinte.159.13.1473.

Willy, U., Mohamed, B., Eric, S., Andrew, S., Kisali, P., Ephraim, M.,

Fred, M. and **Gunnel, B. 2004:** Rate of decline of absolute number and percentage of CD4 T-lymphocytes among HIV-1 infected adults in Dar es Salaam, Tanzania. *AIDS*. Vol.18 (3): 433-438.

WHO 1981: Intestinal protozoan and helminthic infection. Report of WHO scientific group, WHO Tech Rep Ser. 666.

WHO 1985: http://www.who.int

WHO 1987: Technical Report Series, 749.

WHO 1996: http://www.who.int

WHO 1999: World Health Report, 1999 (http://www.who.int)

WHO 2001: Guidelines on standard operating procedures for laboratory diagnosis of HIV opportunistic infections. New Delhi, India.

WHO 2003a: Bench Aids for the diagnosis of intestinal parasites, Reprinted copy, Geneva.

WHO 2003b: Manual of basic techniques for a health laboratory, 2nd Edition, Geneva ISBN 92 4 1545305.

WHO 2010: A summary of evidence for the revised WHO principles and recommendations on HIV and infant feeding. Geneva, World Health Organisation.

Wolday, D., Mayaan, S., Mariam, Z.G., Berhe, Seboxe, T., Britton, S., Galai, N., Landay, A. and Bentwich, Z. 2002: Treatment of intestinal worm is associated with decreased HIV plasma viral load. *J Acq Immun Defic Syndr*. 31: 56-62.

Wong, M.S. and **Bundy, D.A.P. 1990:** Quantitative assessment of contamination of soil by the eggs of *Ascaris lumbricoides* and *Trichuris trichiura. Trans R Soc Trop Med Hyg* 84, 567 – 570.

Xiao, L., Lal, R.B. and **Lal, A.A. 1999**: Effect of immune activation induced by *Cryptosporidium parvum* whole antigen on in vitro human immunodeficiency virus type 1 infection. *J Infect Dis*. 180, 559 - 563.

Zida, A., Yacouba, A., Sawadogo, M. P., Diallo, I., Sangare, I., Bamba, S., Ouattara, B. and **Guiguemde, D. R. (2017)**: Opportunistic and other intestinal parasites infection among HIV-positive patients in the era of combination antiretroviral therapy and preventive treatment in Ouagadougou, Burkina Faso. *J HIV Clin Sci Res* 4 (2): 008 – 0014, DOI: http://doi.org/10.17352/2455-3786.000122.

Zope, A., Pai, A., De, A. and **Baveja, M. 2014**: Opportunistic intestinal parasites in HIV infected individuals and its correlation with the CD4 counts. *Resh & Rev: J Med Hlth Sc* 3(4): Jul – Sept 2014, 55 -60.

PHOTO PLATES

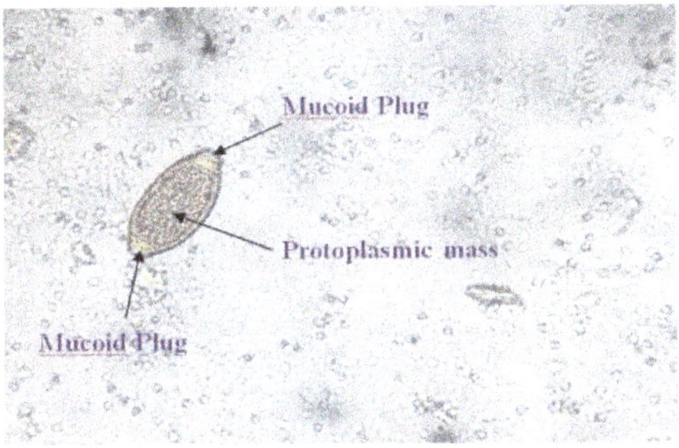

Bile stained barrel shaped egg of *Trichuris trichiura* (40x) [Ethyl acetate concentration technique]

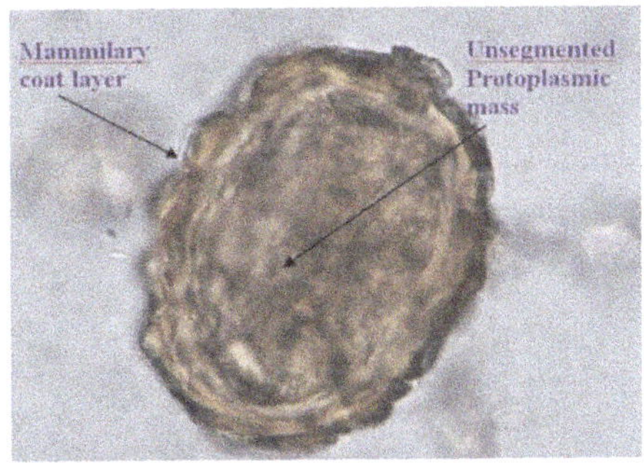

Fertilized corticated egg of *Ascaris lumbricoides* (40x) [Ethyl acetate concentration technique]

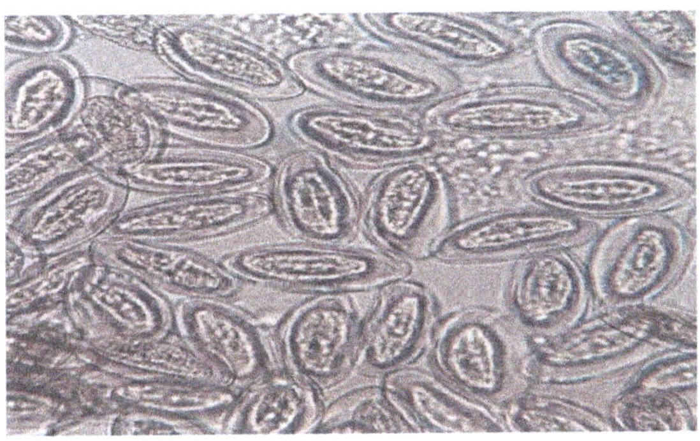

Partially embryonated plano convex egg of *Enterobius vermicularis* (40x) [Adhesive cellophane tape method]

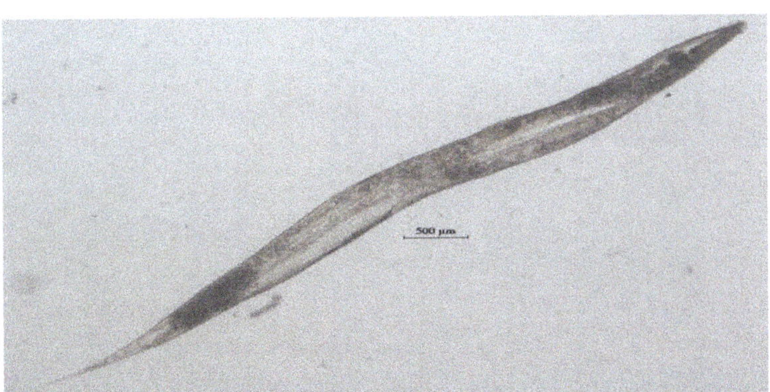

♀ *Enterobius vermicularis* W.M. (8x) [Scrapping with a soft brush from the peri anal region]

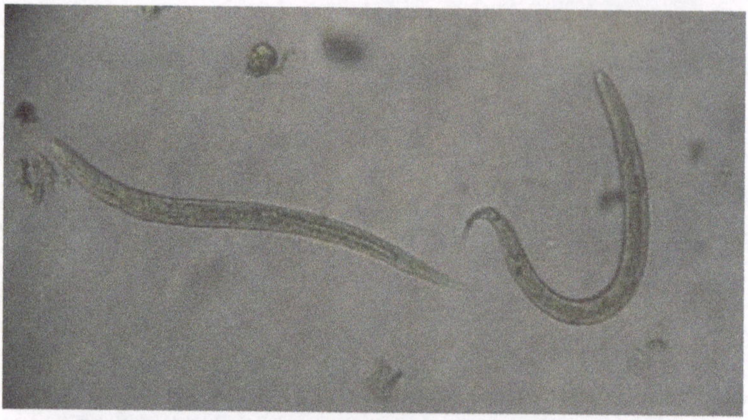

Rhabditiform larvae of hookworm (10x) [Ethyl acetate concentration technique]

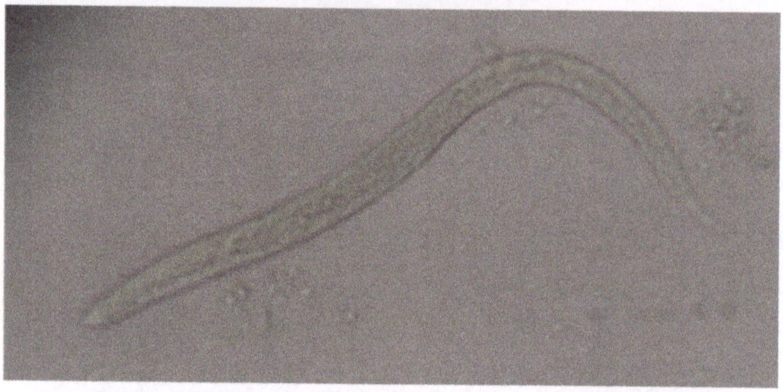

Rhabditiform larva of *Strongyloides stercoralis* (40x) [Modified Baermann funnel technique]

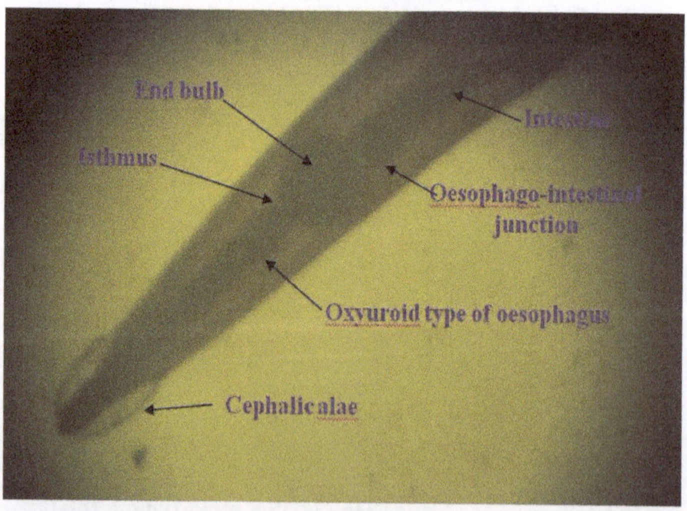

Anterior end of *Enterobius vermicularis* showing the oxyuroid type of oesophagus, isthmus, cephalic alae, end bulb and oesophago-intestinal junction (40x)

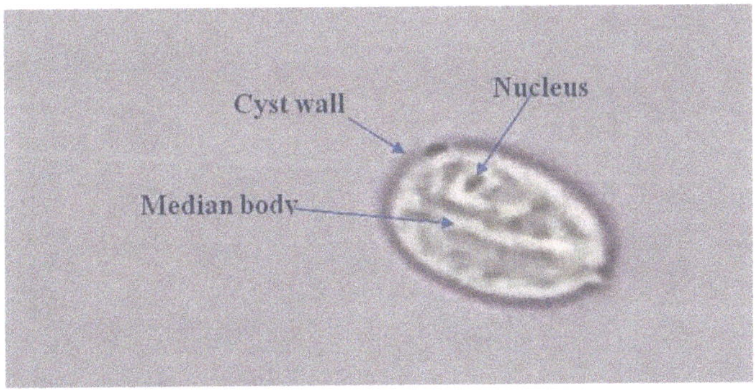

Cyst of *Giardia lamblia* (40x) [Ethyl acetate concentration technique]

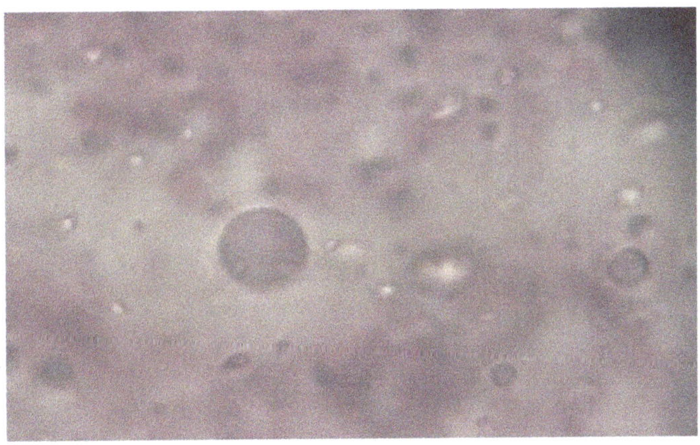

Cyst of *Entamoeba histolytica* (40x) [Ethyl acetate concentration technique]

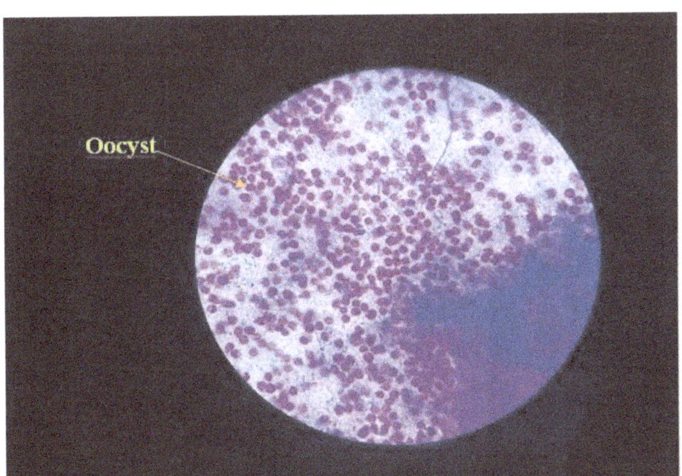

Oocyst of *Cryptosporidium* (100x) Modified Ziehl Neelsen staining technique

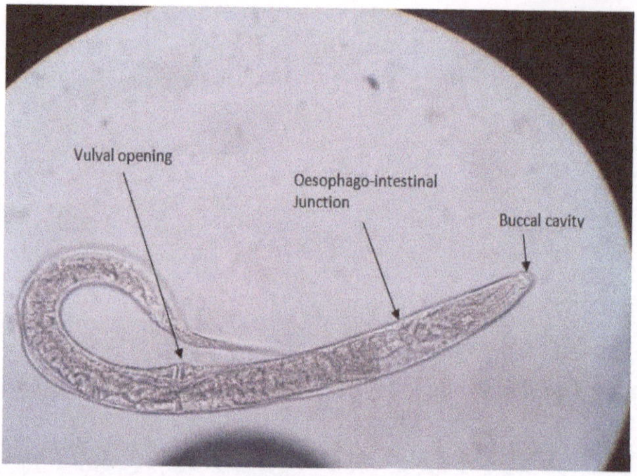

Strongyloides stercoralis **(Female, 40x) After treatment with normal saline, physiological saline, PBS, & GA**

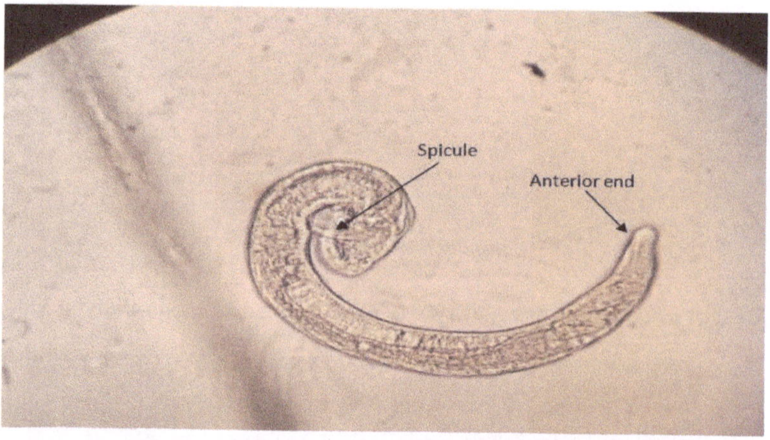

Strongyloides stercoralis **(Male, 40x) After treatment with normal saline, physiological saline, PBS & GA**

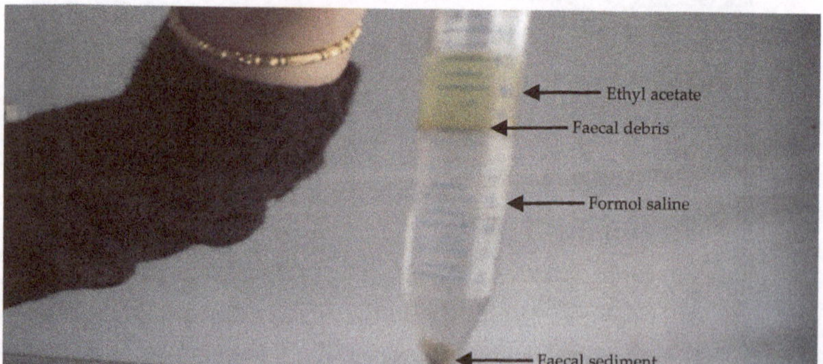

Showing the presence of four layers in a centrifuge tube when the sample is subjected to Ethyl acetate concentration technique

Printed at Repro India Ltd.